Vasoplegic Endothelial Dysfunction

Paulo Roberto Barbosa Evora
Andrea Carla Celotto
Agnes Afrodite Sumarelli Albuquerque
Patricia Martinez Évora

Vasoplegic Endothelial Dysfunction

Circulatory Shock and Methylene Blue

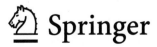 Springer

Paulo Roberto Barbosa Evora
Department of Surgery and Anatomy
Ribeirão Preto Medical School/ USP
Ribeirão Preto, São Paulo
Brazil

Agnes Afrodite Sumarelli Albuquerque
Department of Surgery and Anatomy
Ribeirão Preto Medical School/ USP
Ribeirão Preto, São Paulo
Brazil

Andrea Carla Celotto
Ribeirão Preto Medical School/ USP
Ribeirão Preto, São Paulo
Brazil

Patricia Martinez Évora
Ribeirão Preto Medical School/ USP
Ribeirão Preto, São Paulo
Brazil

Original Portuguese edition published by Editora Atheneu Ltda., São Paulo, Brazil, 2011
ISBN 978-3-030-74098-6   ISBN 978-3-030-74096-2   (eBook)
https://doi.org/10.1007/978-3-030-74096-2

This Springer imprint is published by the registered company Springer Nature Switzerland AG
The registered company address is: Gewerbestrasse 11, 6330 Cham, Switzerland

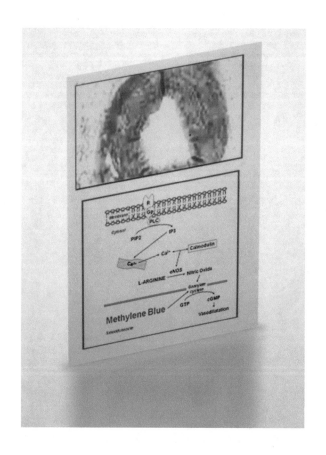

A book dedication is a way for authors to honor a person (or a group of people) they would like to thank, and usually is/are not one of the authors. However, this dedication will "break protocols" to honor the one who taught us to do so at opportune times: Dr. Paulo Evora, affectionately called PE by his former, yet eternal students. We dedicate this book to you, PE, the great creator of this work, who, in addition to being a surgeon, intensivist, and researcher of excellence, has qualities that make one a special human being: humanization, empathy, kindness, generosity, sensitivity, tenderness, and very good mood. You were, are, and always will be our true master because your teachings go far beyond science, they are true life lessons, and your attitudes are always good examples. Thank you for being our scientific father and for making this paternal relationship go beyond the limits of the laboratory, never being too busy to help, let alone resting until any issue is completely resolved. Thank you for sharing and instigating us to seek knowledge with respect, dedication, and passion. Thank you for teaching us, in practice, the real meaning and importance of collective work and for brilliantly leading the "endothelium squad," which was unbeatable in academic-scientific missions. Thank you for, in the moments when everything seemed to be going wrong, comforting us and reminding us that life and research are a mix of "days of euphoria and days of depression." Thank you for each tear accompanied by a trembling pout of cry in our defenses; your sensitivity taught us to let emotions show. Thank you for stimulating our creative potential and expanding our horizons through your "serendipity." Thank you for encouraging us to "fatten the capybara" (a PE slang for curriculum improvement) and to "distribute our eggs in several baskets"; these incentives were essential for us to fly in other directions, but without ever forgetting our principles and our trajectory, which, scientifically, started in the "endothelium squad" and still remains united in friendship, respect, and admiration for you. Finally, it is impossible to describe in this space everything we have learned in these several years of working with you, PE, but we would like you to know that we are immensely grateful that you are part of our lives, and that we will continue to do our best, always remembering that "the great is the enemy of the good." "Kisses" and "huggies" from the "endothelium squad"! This dedication was written by the authors Andréa, Agnes, and Patricia, with the contribution of former students Luciana,

Fernanda, and Verena. It symbolizes gratitude to the great master Dr. Paulo Roberto Barbosa Evora from all the students who experienced the Endothelial Function Laboratory.[1]

---

[1] Words and expressions highlighted in quotation marks are those that Dr. Paulo Evora often said in our conversations.

Foreword

Cardiovascular surgeons have long appreciated the importance and central role of vascular endothelium in maintaining vessel patency and tone and in vascular remodeling in response to stress and injury. The discoveries of vasoactive factors released by endothelial cells have provided mechanisms for understanding local and systemic effects of the endothelium which functions as an endocrine organ. Indeed, in humans, the total weight of several trillion vascular endothelial cells may be as great as 1 kg, making the surface of arteries and veins one of the largest endocrine organs in the body, second only to the gut.

In this book, the authors have leveraged Dr. Evora's experience as a clinical surgeon and his many contributions from the experimental laboratory to educate the reader in endothelial cell physiology and pathophysiology. The 17 chapters are organized into 4 parts. Each chapter begins with an abstract and ends with selected references; especially helpful are the "Concluding Remarks" which succinctly summarize the important concepts with bullet points.

Chapter 1 reviews basic aspects of mediators released by the endothelium including relaxing factors and contracting factors. This part might be considered required reading for clinicians who deal with cardiovascular disease. The molecular mechanisms controlling synthesis and release of vasoactive factors from the endothelium are thoroughly discussed, and the chapter ends with the important concept of "constitutive" forms of nitric oxide synthase, which depend on $Ca2+$ and calmodulin release, and inducible nitric oxide synthase, which can be induced by cytokines and is upregulated in many systemic disorders.

In Part 2, the authors give an overview of shock states and ischemia/reperfusion. They use the practical classification of hypovolemic, cardiogenic, obstructive, and distributive shock and discuss mechanisms of organ failure as well as ischemia/ reperfusion injury. The authors correctly emphasize the importance of correcting the underlying cause of shock but also introduce the notion that circulatory collapse due to vasoplegia, as can occur with sepsis, anaphylaxis, and other systemic inflammatory states, is likely mediated, at least in part, by the endothelium through excess production of nitric oxide. This understanding is the basis for subsequent discussions of the use of methylene blue as an adjunct in the management of vaso-plegia, an area of special interest of Dr. Evora and his team.

Most physicians know of methylene blue as a dye that is useful in treating met-hemoglobinemia, but as discussed in Part 3, methylene blue is a potent inhibitor of guanylate cyclase, a target enzyme in the endothelium-dependent relaxation medi-ated by nitric oxide. Methylene blue has been found to be very effective in improv-ing arterial blood pressure. Chapters in this part describe several additional conditions in which the inhibitory effect of methylene blue on nitric oxide produc-tion may be useful, including burn injury, neuroprotection following cardiac arrest, and management of vasoplegia during and after cardiopulmonary bypass. This last area is particularly important to cardiac surgeons and anesthesiologists as post bypass vasoplegia is recognized more commonly now than in the earlier days of cardiac surgery. Risk factors for postoperative vasoplegia include preoperative use of heparin, ACE inhibitors, congestive heart failure, poor left ventricular function, prolonged duration of cardiopulmonary bypass, and opioid anesthesia. Dr. Evora and his team have pioneered the use of methylene blue for postoperative vasoplegia, which can be especially difficult to manage in patients undergoing cardiac surgery for active endocarditis. The use of methylene blue allows lower doses of other vaso-constrictors in these critically ill patients. Chapter 13 ends with a useful protocol for use of methylene blue during cardiopulmonary bypass. Additional important detail on the use of methylene blue is covered in Part 4.

Much attention has been given to translational research and laboratory investiga-tion that leads to improvements in patient outcomes. The clinical studies of Dr. Evora on methylene blue are directly related to his extensive laboratory investiga-tions of endothelial function and pharmacology, and are excellent examples of "bench to bedside." I know he joins me in hoping that this book, which nicely sum-marizes his efforts and interests, will stimulate other young investigators to extend the study of endothelial function, both basic research and rigorous clinical trials of medications such as methylene blue.

Hartzell V. Schaff
Department of Cardiovascular Surgery
Mayo Clinic
Rochester, MN, USA

Preface

Why is methylene blue (MB) the only option for blocking the cgmp/no pathway in the treatment of vasoplegic shock (VS)? "Reasons that reason itself does not know..."

There is no evidence of the word shock being used in its modern-day form before 1743. However, there is evidence that Hippocrates used the word *exemia* to signify a state of being "drained of blood." Shock or "choc" was first described in a trauma victim in the English translation of Henri-François LeDran's 1740 text, "Traité ou Reflexions Tire'es de la Pratique sur les Playes d'armes à feu" (a treatise, or reflections, drawn from practice on gun-shot wounds.) In this text, he describes "choc" as a reaction to the sudden impact. However, the first English writer to use the word shock in its modern-day connotation was James Latta in 1795 [1].

George W. Crile, in 1899, suggested in his monograph, *An Experimental Research into Surgical Shock,* that shock was a state of circulatory collapse due to excessive nervous stimulation. Other competing theories around the turn of the century included one penned by Malcolm in 1905. The assertion was that prolonged vasoconstriction led to the pathophysiological signs and symptoms of shock. Following World War I, research around shock resulted in experiments by Walter B. Cannon at Harvard and William M. Bayliss at London in 1919, which showed that an increase in permeability of the capillaries in response to trauma or toxins was responsible for many clinical manifestations of shock. In 1972, Hinshaw and Cox suggested a shock classification system, which is still used today [1].

Perhaps the best approach to defining the state of shock is that of Robert Hardaway, who begins his discussion by stating, "What shock is not." This approach is interesting because it demonstrates the entire evolution of circulatory shock as the pathophysiological concepts have changed. Thus, the shock is not: (1) low blood pressure – due to the hypothalamus-pituitary-adrenal axis (release of catecholamines and cortisol) normal and even supranormal blood pressure can be maintained; (2) a low pH does not necessarily accompany it – it can be normal or even alkalotic depending on the endogenous production of bicarbonate and the compensatory hyperventilation to metabolic acidosis; (3) it is not always accompanied by low cardiac output – there are hyperdynamic states associated, for example, with sepsis; (4) it is not due to the exhaustion of the adrenal gland – in pre-death, plasma levels of catecholamines are high; (5) arteriolodilatation does not necessarily exist – the rule is that vasoconstriction occurs; and (6) there is not necessarily hypovolemia – an example is a cardiogenic shock resulting from acute myocardial infarction. After these considerations, it would remain to define "what shock is," and, in search of a universal definition, it was concluded that the best definition of the shock state would be: "inadequate capillary perfusion" or, simply, "bad tissue perfusion." These concepts are from the 1970s and are linked to the Vietnam War.

The discovery and the massive NO scientific investment annulled paradigms, starting a new era of knowledge. Vasoplegia associated with systemic inflammatory reaction to the condition of "enemy to be overcome." The concepts emerging from the observations obtained during the first 15 years of using MB for VS treatment in cardiac surgery have established some critical topics. But, we still feel that the cGMP's importance is underestimated in the literature [5].

In 2009, we published a personal statement centered at MB as a treatment of VS in cardiac surgery, including 15 years of questions, answers, doubts, and certainties [2]. Some repetitive observations can be applied to VS: (1) MB is safe at the recommended doses (the lethal dose is 40 mg.Kg^{-1}); (2) the use of MB does not cause endothelial dysfunction; (3) the MB effect appears in cases of positive NO regulation; (4) MB itself is not a vasoconstrictor, because by blocking the cGMP pathway, it releases the adenosine 3'5' – cyclic monophosphate (cAMP) pathway, facilitating the vasoconstrictor effect of epinephrine; (5) the MB may act through this mechanism of "crosstalk," and its use as a medication of the first choice may not be correct; (6) the most used dosage is 2 mg.Kg^{-1} in IV bolus, followed by the same continuous doses infusion because the plasma concentrations decrease markedly in the first 40 minutes. Although there are no definitive multicenter studies, the MB used in the treatment of VS cardiac surgery is currently the best, safest, and cheapest option; however, a possible 'window of opportunity for the effectiveness of MB is not established for humans.

This editorial has the primary purpose of performing a simple exercise of logic. The following are well established [3, 4]:

1. The inflammatory reaction is present in all types of circulatory shock.
2. If vasoplegia is present for a long time, a "vasoplegic endothelial dysfunction" with catecholamine-resistant arterial hypotension leads irreversibly to death.
3. This dysfunction is mediated by the cGMP/NO system and its blocking by Methylene Blue.
4. Currently, the blockage of sGC by MB, despite the most varied criticisms, and despite MB being the first drug used in humans over 100 years ago, is still a matter of controversy.

What is the basis for the proposed logic exercise?

The NO pathway blocking is already part of the vasoplegia therapeutic arsenal. However, assuming that the MB is at least controversial, why isn't there any investment in discovering an alternative drug? Restrictions on MB can be disguised as a mandatory objective. From the physiological point of view, a bias toward the blockage of the cGMP/NO pathway hides its fundamental importance. In other words, the resistance to MB use can blunt this importance. ***Therefore, why isn't there a search for an alternative MB drug?***

Finally, even though Blaise Pascoal once said "Reasons That Reason Itself does not know ...?", science and pharmaceutical industry are in debt.

References

1. Saha BK, Burns SL. The story of nitric oxide, sepsis and methylene blue: a comprehensive pathophysiologic review. Am J Med Sci. 2020;360(4):329–37. https://doi.org/10.1016/j.amjms.2020.06.007. Epub 2020 Jun 6. PMID: 32631574.
2. Evora PR, Ribeiro PJ, Vicente WV, Reis CL, Rodrigues AJ, Menardi AC, et al. Methylene blue for vasoplegic syndrome treatment in heart surgery: fifteen years of questions, answers, doubts and certainties. Rev Bras Cir Cardiovasc. 2009;24(3):279–88.
3. Evora PR. An open discussion about endothelial dysfunction: is it timely to propose a classification? Int J Cardiol. 2000;73(3):289–92.
4. Evora PR, Alves Junior L, Ferreira CA, Menardi AC, Bassetto S, Rodrigues AJ, et al. Twenty years of vasoplegic syndrome treatment in heart surgery. Methylene blue revised. Rev Bras Cir Cardiovasc. 2015;30(1):84–92.
5. Shanmugam G. Vasoplegic syndrome- the role of methylene blue. Eur J Cardiothorac Surg. 2005;28(5):705–10.

Acknowledgments

To the research foundations for the constant funding of our clinical and experimental investigations

- São Paulo Research Foundation (FAPESP)
- National Council of Scientific and Technological Development (CNPq)
- Coordination of Improvement of Higher Academic Staff (CAPES)
- Support for Teaching, Research and Assistance at HCFMRP-USP (FAEPA)

To Springer Nature for editorial support based on professionalism and dedication

- Vanessa Shimabukuro
- Janakiraman Ganesan
- ArulRonika Pathinathan

Contents

Part I
General Conceptual Aspects

Chapter 1
Introduction

Currently, the endothelium is considered an organ that performs numerous metabolic functions, participating in the regulation of vascular tone. This regulation uses several mechanisms (metabolic, myogenic, and neuroendocrine); in fact, there is an essential interaction between all these mechanisms. The endothelium is responsible for the paracrine regulation of the vascular tone, emphasizing the scientific impact of the establishment of nitric oxide (NO) as a vasodilator and endogenous anti-thrombotic [1].

In 1980, Furchgott and Zawadzki discovered a fact that for many years was a great pharmacology enigma: Acetylcholine in some situations is a vasoconstrictor, and in others, it acts as a vasodilator. The simple verification that acetylcholine only acts as a vasodilator in the presence of the endothelium triggered an era of intense work in the 1980s, which established the endothelium as the site of the triggering of most cardiovascular diseases [2].

It was postulated, then, the existence of an endothelium-derived relaxing factor which, in 1982, was called the endothelium-derived relaxing factor (EDRF). In these pioneering studies, it was determined that EDRF was not a prostanoid, since indomethacin, a blocker of the cyclooxygenase pathway, did not inhibit endothelium-dependent relaxation, produced by acetylcholine and many other agonists, such as ADP, serotonin, histamine, and many others. It was also determined that EDRF was diffusible and dependent on calcium ions.

A significant contribution, from a scientific point of view, occurred in 1985 when Cocks and Angus were able to grow endothelial cells and install them in a perfusion circuit that allowed obtaining large amounts of EDRF for biochemical and pharmacological manipulation [3].

It was discovered, then, that endothelium-dependent relaxation was associated with an increase in cGMP in vascular smooth muscle, which can be inhibited by methylene blue (MB) and hemoglobin ("sequester" or EDRF scavenger). It was also discovered that EDRF could be destroyed by superoxide anions and other free radicals, supporting the concept that EDRF, by itself, was a radical. With the

© The Author(s), under exclusive license to Springer Nature Switzerland AG 2021
P. R. Barbosa Evora et al., *Vasoplegic Endothelial Dysfunction*,
https://doi.org/10.1007/978-3-030-74096-2_1

accumulation of evidence that EDRF had many of the nitrovasodilators characteristics, Furchgott and Ignarro independently proposed, at the IV symposium on "vasodilation mechanisms" held at the Mayo Clinic in 1986, that EDRF was NO. The research was then directed towards determining how the endothelium produced the radical and culminated in the proposition of Palmer and Moncada, who postulated that L-arginine was the source of NO under the action of an enzyme, nitric oxide synthase [4].

> The normal state of the cardiovascular system is that of constant and active vasodilation. If this is true, then we will have to review normal cardiovascular physiology, taking this vasodilator tone into account. In addition, in the coming years we will have to review some of our concepts of pathophysiology. We will probably even have to change the name of some conditions; for example, hypertension can best be described as hypovasodilation.

This quote is classic and defines clearly what the discovery of EDRF/NO represented in the international scientific scenario. Studies from the 1990s definitively established the role of the endothelium in all cardiovascular diseases, which were associated with endothelial dysfunction due to impaired release of endothelium-derived relaxing factors with a consequent risk of spasm and thrombosis.

Injury or activation of the endothelium modifies its regulatory functions resulting in abnormal function. Endothelial dysfunction has been defined as an imbalance between relaxing and contracting factors, pro-coagulation mediators, and anticoagulants or between inhibitory and growth-promoting substances. Clinically, the "syndrome" of endothelial dysfunction can be described as local or generalized vasospasm, thrombosis, atherosclerosis, and restenosis. It is interesting to note that most of the texts on endothelial dysfunction associate its presence with the impairment of the release of vasoactive endothelial substances without considering the vasoplegia caused by the more significant version of these vasorelaxant factors. This fact motivated us to propose an open discussion about the desirability of classifying endothelial dysfunction [1–3].

The decrease in systemic vascular resistance observed in irreversible hypovolemic shock, septic shock, and vasoplegias associated with systemic inflammatory reactions and anaphylaxis is associated with excessive NO production. In these situations, NO induces loss of vascular sensitivity to catecholamines and myocardial depression, contributing to lethal hypotension. Any process in which pro-inflammatory cytokines are released can cause excess NO production as occurs, eventually, in patients undergoing cardiopulmonary bypass. Clinical studies also show an increase in NO production in adults and children with different forms of shock, with increased serum nitrate correlated with systemic vasodilation.

Vessels isolated from animals in shock show a pronounced hyporeactivity to practically all tested vasoconstrictor agents (adrenaline, norepinephrine, phenylephrine, dopamine, endothelin, angiotensin, thromboxane, etc.). NOS inhibitors and specific iNOS inhibitors can reverse this hyporeactivity. Although endothelial cells can be induced to form NO, the significant production source may be the smooth muscle of the vessel itself. NO produced by iNOS expression within the vasculature is responsible for excessive vasodilation and reduced contractile responses to vaso-constrictor agents.

In addition to data demonstrating an increased formation of NO by iNOS in various forms of shock, there are convincing data that show the impairment of NO biosynthesis by the ecNOS expression in the vascular endothelium in situations of hemorrhagic or endotoxic shock. This mechanism is sometimes referred to as a functional exchange between NOS isoforms, with the iNOS expression and ecNOS infra-regulation at the same time. The impairment of ecNOS expression can be harmful to essential organs such as the brain, heart, and kidneys, thus associating with multiple organ dysfunctions. The reduction of NO production is also related to antiplatelet activity and activation of polymorphonuclear leukocytes, contributing, by peroxynitrite-dependent mechanisms, to endothelial and tissue damage.

From a hemodynamic point of view, the cardiocirculatory shock can be classified into three groups: (1) primary or secondary myocardial failure, (2) acute volume loss or vascular obstruction, and (3) alteration of vascular capacitance. Although this classification is useful for academic discussions, clinical presentations are much more complicated, with different pathophysiological mechanisms present in the same patient (e.g., septic shock associated with hypovolemia and myocardial depression). In some patients, the onset of symptoms may be delayed due to compensatory mechanisms such as increased cardiac output and catecholamines release. Although most shock states are associated with decreased cardiac output, a different situation occurs in cases of shocks due to reduced vascular capacitance. In these cases, the vasoplegia is associated with increased cardiac output, configuring a hyperdynamic action with severe hypotension resistant to high doses of catecholamines. It is essential to report that even in this situation, myocardial depression can occur with low ejection fractions and biventricular dilation. The poor prognosis seems to be better correlated with low vascular resistance, leading to the conclusion that vasoplegia is the determining prognostic factor. Thus, paracrine control of vascular capacitance becomes a crucial factor for clinical and experimental investigations in the search for new pathophysiological and therapeutic knowledge that can contribute to the vasoplegia treatment and prognosis. It should be noted that vasoplegic endothelial dysfunction is associated with all types of shock states, which will be addressed in this book.

Proposal for Classification of Endothelial Dysfunction

To facilitate and allow an overview of endothelial dysfunction, we proposed a classification. This is the only existing classification, but curiously we were not able to start an open discussion on the subject [5–7].

(I) *Etiological Classification.* (A) Primary or "genotypic" endothelial dysfunction: demonstrated in homozygous children with homocystinuria and in normotensive patients with a family history of essential arterial hypertension. (B) Secondary or "phenotypic" endothelial dysfunction: present in all cardiovascular diseases (atherosclerosis, coronary heart disease, high blood pressure, diabetes, and others).
(II) *Functional Classification.* (A) "Vasotonic" endothelial dysfunction: present in cardiovascular diseases, which implies a risk of vasospasm and thrombosis. (B) "Vasoplegic" endothelial dysfunction: present in distributive shock states caused by cytokine actions that stimulate the pathological release of relaxing endothelial factors, mainly nitric oxide (sepsis, anaphylaxis, anaphylactoid reactions, and vasoplegia related to extracorporeal circulation).
(III) *Evolutive or Prognostic Classification.* (A) "Reversible" endothelial dysfunction: most likely to occur in the early stages of "vasoplegic" dysfunction. (B) "Partly reversible" endothelial dysfunction: to include the idea that it is possible to improve endothelial dysfunction without complete reversal. "Vasotonic" dysfunctions associated with cardiovascular diseases are probably impossible to completely reverse. (C) Irreversible endothelial dysfunction: Evolution of cardiovascular diseases and sepsis.

These data, added to the total nonconformity against death, mainly when significant battles are lost against septic shocks in young women with gynecological infections, as well as patients who die from anaphylactic shock, were the primary motivation of a line of research that led to the preparation of this book. It is part of a constant and growing effort to save lives, like that of the people mentioned above, looking for therapeutic alternatives to what we classify as "vasoplegic endothelial dysfunction."

References

1. Evora PR. The scientific impact of the nitric oxide discovery as vasodilator and endogenous antithrombotic agent. Arq Bras Cardiol. 1993;61(1):3–5.
2. Furchgott RF, Zawadzki JV. The obligatory role of endothelial cells in the relaxation of arterial smooth muscle by acetylcholine. Nature. 1980;288(5789):373–6.
3. Cocks TM, Angus JA. Bioassay of the release of EDRF from isolated endothelial cells in vitro. In: Bevan JA, Godfraind T, Maxwell RA, Stoclet JC, Worcel M, editors. Vascular neuroeffector mechanisms. Amsterdam: Elsevier Science Pub; 1984. p. 131–6.
4. Palmer RM, Ferrige AG, Moncada S. Nitric oxide release accounts for the biological activity of endothelium-derived relaxing factor. Nature. 1987;327(6122):524–6.
5. Evora PR. An open discussion about endothelial dysfunction: is it timely to propose a classification? Int J Cardiol. 2000;73(3):289–92.
6. Evora PR, Baldo CF, Celotto AC, Capellini VK. Endothelium dysfunction classification: why is it still an open discussion? Int J Cardiol. 2009;137(2):175–6.
7. Arcencio L, Evora PR. The lack of clinical applications would be the cause of low interest in an endothelial dysfunction classification. Arq Bras Cardiol. 2017;108(2):97–9.

Chapter 2
Physiology of the Endothelium

The endothelium of arteries and veins has long been studied by doctors and researchers who deal with cardiovascular diseases. However, a global view of endothelial function was not possible until the past two decades that witnessed the discovery of prostacyclin production, the subsequent discovery of endothelium-derived nitric oxide (NO), and other vasoactive factors. Far from being a passive interface barrier between blood flow and the body, the endothelium must be considered as an organic system whose function is critical in maintaining blood anticoagulation in vivo, maintaining vascular tone, and regulating perfusion. There are three known endothelium-dependent vasodilation mechanisms: (1) dependent on the cGMP system (NO – nitric oxide); (2) dependent on the adenosine 3'5'-cyclic monophosphate (cAMP) system (PGI_2 – prostacyclin); and (3) hyperpolarization (EDHF – hyperpolarizing factor of the endothelium still unknown or nonexistent) (Fig. 2.1). These mechanisms are synergistic with each other, with NO being the most important factor, because in addition to being an endogenous vasodilator, it is also an antiplatelet factor [1–3].

Impaired release by endothelial dysfunction creates conditions for spasm and thrombosis, while excess release leads to vasoplegia and a tendency to diffuse bleeding (Fig. 2.2).

Nitric Oxide Release Pathway

There are now a series of events that participate in an "EDRF/NO formation cascade." Taking as an example the endothelium-dependent relaxation induced by acetylcholine (ACh), the pathway description would be ACh stimulates a muscarinic receptor and releases EDRF/NO that spreads to the vascular smooth muscle, causing an increase in guanosine 3'5'-cyclic monophosphate (cGMP) with vasodilation. It is only a partial view, since the process is a little more elaborate, involving a

P. R. Barbosa Evora et al., *Vasoplegic Endothelial Dysfunction*, https://doi.org/10.1007/978-3-030-74096-2_2

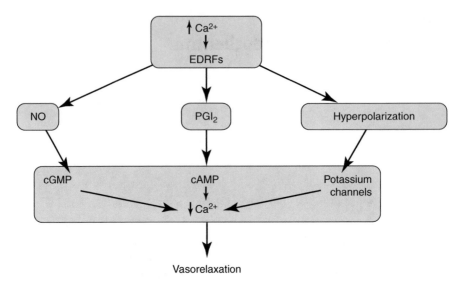

Fig. 2.1 Vasodilation mechanisms. Ca^{2+} calcium, EDRFs endothelium-derived relaxing factor, NO nitric oxide, PGI_2 prostacyclin, cGMP guanosine 3′5′-cyclic monophosphate, cAMP adenosine 3′5′-cyclic monophosphate

transduction system with secondary messengers that include G-proteins, which make the connection with the phosphatidylinositol pathway, which, in turn, mobilizes the intracellular calcium necessary for the formation of NO from L-arginine by the action of nitric oxide synthase (NOS). This cascade of events is far from definitive, which is why researchers from various parts of the world have endeavored to discover pharmacological "markers" for the study of the multiple steps of the classic pathway for the release of EDRF/NO, all of which may have a participation in the genesis of cardiovascular diseases [1–3].

Alterations at the level of receptors are studied by several agonists, with ACh being widely used as a neurotransmitter stimulating muscarinic receptors and ADP as a platelet product. Regarding the signal transduction between receptors and intracellular processes, although not yet entirely accepted as a definitive marker, numerous experiments suggest that sodium fluoride produces endothelium-dependent relaxation, through a pathway that is sensitive to pertussis toxin. The "tool" to study the phosphatidylinositol pathway is phospholipase C, emphasizing its specificity since phospholipases B and D do not induce endothelium-dependent vasodilation. The synergism between EDRF/NO and prostacyclin may occur via the phosphatidylinositol pathway. Next, the calcium ionophore A23187 deserves to be highlighted, which promotes endothelium-dependent vasodilation, but independent of membrane receptors shows that the endothelial cell maintains the capacity to produce NO.

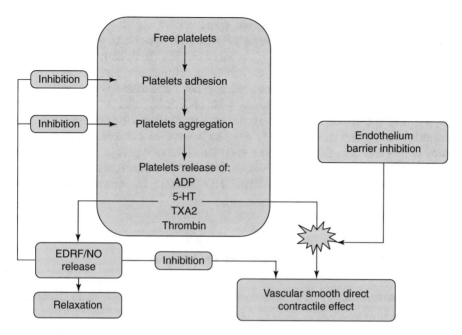

Fig. 2.2 Vasodilator and antiplatelet actions of nitric oxide. EDRFs endothelium-derived relaxing factor, NO nitric oxide

EDRF/NO

The release of EDRF or EDRFs, once the existence of more than one endothelial factor is postulated, can occur through different pathways involving G proteins and independent mechanisms. The G protein is responsible for mediating the inhibitory effects of receptors on the adenyl cyclase pathway. Little is known about the transduction signal, involving the synthesis or release of EDRF/NO. An early stage in most receptor-mediated responses is the activation of G-proteins in the cell membrane, which can initiate the modulation of a variety of intracellular events. The activation of regulatory G proteins is associated with the agonist stimulation of most receptors linked to the cell membrane. Therefore, specific agonist-receptor interactions facilitate the binding of guanine triphosphate to an alpha subunit of the protein, and the G protein is activated. G protein then dissociates from the receptor causing a reduction in the affinity of the receptor for the agonist, and the alpha subunit is released. The distinct alpha subunits derived from different G proteins can activate various intracellular processes [1, 2]. The identity of this(ese) G protein(s) and its(their) relationship to G proteins, involving alpha1-adrenergic stimulation of phospholipase C, is not known. The role of G protein(s) in the pathophysiology of vasospasm after global ischemia and reperfusion is also unclear. Their participation was proven by comparatively studying the vascular relaxations caused by sodium fluoride. This element was able to produce biphasic responses in human, bovine, and pig coronary arteries, specifically causing dependent relaxation and independent endothelium contraction. The dysfunction of these G proteins in the endothelium has also been postulated as responsible for endothelial dysfunction in conditions with endothelial cell regeneration after injury, atherosclerosis, and coronary vasospasm. Although the description of the transduction system mediated by G proteins is somewhat complicated, its inclusion in this text is justified given the enormous scientific perspective of its study in the genesis of cardiovascular diseases. It should be noted that it participates in signal transduction, not only in EDRF/NO but also in several other mediators [1–3].

Agonists of the Nitric Oxide Release Pathway

The system involved in the NO release can be studied using its agonists and receptors (Fig. 2.3) [3].

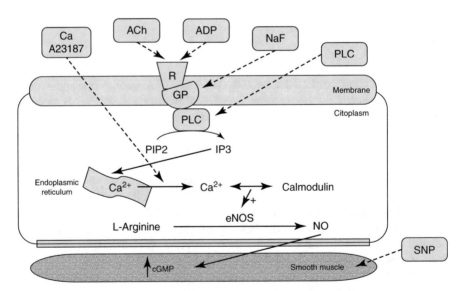

Fig. 2.3 Nitric oxide release pathway by the endothelial cell and some of its primary pharmacological agonists. CA A23187 calcium ionophore, ACh acetylcholine, ADP adenosine diphosphate, NaF sodium fluoride, PLC phospholipase C, R receptor, Gp G protein, PIP2 phosphatidylinositol 4,5-biphosphate, IP3 inositol triphosphate, Ca²⁺ calcium, NO nitric oxide, cGMP guanosine 3′5′-cyclic monophosphate, eNOS endothelial nitric oxide synthase, NPS sodium nitroprusside

Nitric Oxide Blockers

Other essential elements for the pharmacological study of endothelial function are the blockers of the effects and synthesis of EDRF/NO. Among them, the most important are methylene blue (block at the level of cGMP); hemoglobin (or EDRF/NO scavenger); and the nitric (N^G-nitro-L-arginine, L-NOARG) and methylated (N^G-monomethyl-L-arginine, L-NMMA) forms of L-arginine which are NOS blockers. As the methylated and nitric forms of L-arginine block the oxide nitric synthase by competition, the addition of a large concentration of L-arginine reverses the enzyme block, which does not occur with D-arginine, proving the specificity of L-arginine. In laboratory practice, the enzyme block reversal by the addition of L-arginine is more evident in experiments with L-NMMA (Fig. 2.4) [3].

Contractile Factors Derived from the Endothelium

Although not as well-known and often not considered as necessary as the relaxing factors, the endothelium produces at least four "families" of endothelium-derived contracting factors (EDCFs), in balance with the endothelial vasodilating factors. These contractile factors can be classified into EDCF 1s – factors dependent on the

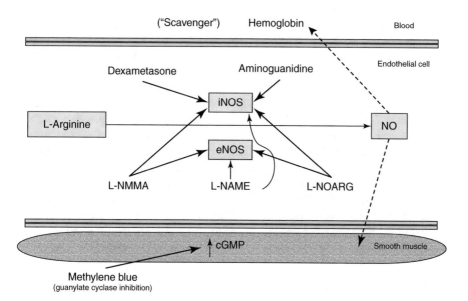

Fig. 2.4 Nitric oxide synthase blockers. *NO* nitric oxide, *cGMP* guanosine 3′5′-cyclic monophosphate, *eNOS* endothelial nitric oxide synthase, *iNOS* inducible nitric oxide synthase, *L-NMMA* N^G-monomethyl-L-arginine, *L-NAME* N^G-nitro-L-arginine methyl ester, *L-NOARG* N^G-nitro-L-arginine

cyclooxygenase pathway; EDCF 2s – the family of endothelins that are vasocon-strictor polypeptides; EDCF 3s – vasoconstrictors released during hypoxia; and EDCF 4s – oxygen-free radicals independent of the cyclooxygenase pathway (Table 2.1) [3].

Currently, there are clear evidences that NO is significant in progressive vasodilation that is associated with various forms of shock. NO is a diatomic gas radical with a noticeably short half-life, which is formed from L-arginine by the expression of a group of enzymes called NOS (Table 2.2). It activates soluble guanylate cyclase, which decreases intracellular calcium and facilitates the relaxation of vascular smooth muscle. Constitutive NOS (ecNOS) usually is present in the vascular endothelium and produces the NO responsible for maintaining vascular tone. An inducible form of NOS (iNOS) is expressed in response to pro-inflammatory stimuli in numerous cells. This enzyme can form NO at a rate up to 1000 times greater than the formation of NO-mediated by ecNOS. iNOS induction is seen in various forms of circulatory shock. In the vascular system, the iNOS expression and a large NO amount produced by this enzyme lead to progressive vasodilation and reduction of blood flow to metabolically active areas, producing organic damage. NO and its reactive product, peroxynitrite, can also cause metabolic inhibition of tissues through various direct cytotoxic mechanisms, such as inhibition of mitochondrial respiration and inactivation of membrane pumps. In addition to progressive vasodilation and metabolic inhibition, the increased formation and release of NO in shock can lead to myocardial depression, although experimental verification is fraught with controversy in this regard. NO-mediated vasodilation and cytotoxicity can be reduced by different pharmacological approaches, including inhibition of NO synthase enzyme activity, NO sequestrators, and guanylate cyclase inhibition. It is expected that the vascular tone restoration will improve physiological changes, with beneficial effects on organic function. This concept can be the first step towards a multiagent therapeutic association for shock states.

Recent data evolving NO synthases are worth mentioning. The so-called "constitutive" (cNOS) forms depend on Ca^{2+} and calmodulin and release picomolar NO concentrations in seconds. The "inducible" (iNOS) is regulated at a pre-transcriptional level and induced by inflammatory cytokines such as tumor necrosis factor-α, interferon-γ, and interleukin-1β and results in the synthesis of large amounts of NO on average 6 hours after exposure to the inflammatory agent [1–3].

In endothelial cells, NO is produced by eNOS, which is involved in the cardiovascular homeostasis control, including blood pressure regulation and cardiac contractility. Signaling for eNOS activation occurs from multiple extracellular stimuli. This enzyme activity depends on the intracellular increase of Ca^{2+}, depletion

Table 2.1 Contractile factors of the endothelium

Endothelium contract factors
EDCF1s – factors dependent on the cyclooxygenase pathway
EDCF2s – endothelin family
EDCF3s – vasoconstrictors released by hypoxia
EDCF4s – oxygen free radicals independent of the cyclooxygenase pathway

Table 2.2 Isoforms of nitric oxide synthases

NO synthases
eNOS – endothelial, physiological, and calcium dependent
nNOS – neuronal, physiological, and calcium dependent
iNOS – inducible, stimulated, and calcium dependent

of the intracellular stocks of Ca^{2+}, and the capacity of its entry through the plasma membrane. eNOS is present in soluble form in the intracellular medium and in the caveolae, where they interact with caveolin-1 while remaining inactive. Caveolae are specialized microdomains found in the plasma membrane of most cells. Studies indicate that there are a variety of molecules organized in the caveolae where they interact to initiate specific signaling cascades. Among these molecules are G protein receptor, IP3 receptor, Ca^{2+}-ATPase, eNOS, arginine transporter (CAT1), and several PKC isoforms.

The eNOS activation present in the caveolae is induced by an increase in the intracellular concentration of Ca^{2+} which promotes the dissociation between eNOS and caveolin-1, thus allowing the complex to bind [2, 3].

There are several mechanisms involved in the entry and exit of calcium from the endothelial cell. Studies have shown that a significant increase in the subplasmalemma concentration of Ca^{2+} may be sufficient for the eNOS activation even in the absence of changes in the perinuclear concentration of Ca^{2+}, suggesting that the focal elevation in the subplasmalemma, more than an overall increase, is the trigger for the NO biosynthesis in the endothelial cell.

The subplasmalemma concentration of Ca^{2+} depends mainly on the plasma membrane Ca^{2+} -ATPase and the Na^+/Ca^{2+} exchanger (NCX). This transporter was first identified in a cardiac cell and carried Na^+ into the cell and Ca^{2+} out, but when it operates in the reverse mode, it transports Ca^{2+} in and Na^+ out.

In the endothelial cell, the presence of NCX was demonstrated by immunohistochemistry and immunofluorescence techniques and cDNA for NCX. Studies also suggest that NCX participates in endothelium-dependent relaxation in arteries by increasing the intracellular concentration of Ca^{2+} when activated in reverse mode.

There is a growing number of studies correlating the NOS activation in the endothelial cell. However, there are still doubts as to how different stimuli activate the signaling pathway that involves such cellular components. In the last 10 years, endothelial glycocalyx has gained considerable importance.

Glycocalyx

The endothelial glycocalyx forms a protective layer of glycosaminoglycans and proteoglycans with adsorbed plasma proteins that cover the endothelial surface. Among its functions, we can mention the vascular permeability regulation, coagulation, and interactions between endothelial cells and circulating blood, acting as a shear stress mechanosensor and controlling vascular tone. The volume and biomechanics of the endothelial glycocalyx are regulated by ionic bonding, hydrogen bonding, and hydrophobic – hydrophilic interactions. Degradation of the endothelial glycocalyx leads to endothelial dysfunction, resulting in unbalanced biomechanics, interruptions in the vessel wall and circulating cell interactions, and loss of sensitivity to shear stress [4].

The vascular endothelium is exposed to shear stress and blood pressure. The glycans on endothelial cell surfaces transmit these mechanical stimuli in intracellular signals that modulate the structure (tubulin and alpha-actin) and endothelial functions. The rearrangement of the glycocalyx cytoskeleton results in the relaxation of smooth muscle cells and vasodilation mediated by the NO release. Blood vessels relatively free from water stress have a higher permeability to macromolecules and suffer more significant atherosclerosis. Glycocalyx dysfunction may be the initial event in the atherothrombotic process and may be involved in the fissure of the atherosclerotic plaque and acute coronary syndromes.

Shear stress stimulates NO production. Weinbaum et al. (2003) described the glycocalyx arrangement in which groups of "bush-like" proteoglycans protrude from anchorage points in the cytoskeleton of the endothelial cell [4]. The mechanical distortion of the entire bush generates forces that deform the under-lying cytoskeleton, increasing the eNOS expression, which catalyzes the NO production and increases hydraulic conductivity. Thus, glycocalyx-mediated vasodilation is a purely mechanical phenomenon, separating it from other modes of NO-mediated vasodilation, including dose-receptor interactions and activation of metabolic pathways in endothelial cells. When there is glycocalyx degradation, a shear-dependent blockage of NO production can be observed. Fluid management is still a controversial topic. The pharmacological differences between crystalloids and colloids are still based mainly on the Starling principle. In the past decade, the glycocalyx has received increasing attention as "a new molecular participant in the great fluid debate." Crystalloids pass freely through the glycocalyx, while colloids are retained in the vasculature by this structure. Numerous retrospective studies have reported a survival benefit when a high proportion of fresh frozen plasma and red blood cells was employed during a massive transfusion that can be explained by the protection or regeneration of the glycocalyx. After intravenous fluid therapy, many clinical and research observations can be explained by incorporating the glycocalyx into the Starling principle. The effects of volume loading to preferentially expand the intravascular space in normovolemic patients are negated by the glycocalyx leakage, resulting in increased vascular permeability. Acute hypervolemic hemodilution causes mechanical stress and glycocalyx lesion mediated by natriuretic peptide, and this may explain why fluids administered in this environment are lost mainly in the interstitial space [5, 6].

Concluding Remarks

- There are three known endothelium-dependent vasodilation mechanisms: (1) dependent on the cGMP system (NO – nitric oxide); (2) dependent on the adenosine $3'5'$-cyclic monophosphate (cAMP) system (PGI$_2$ – prostacyclin) and; (3) hyperpolarization (EDHF – hyperpolarizing factor of the endothelium still unknown or nonexistent).
- Acetylcholine (ACh) "cascade of EDRF/NO formation". ACh stimulates a muscarinic receptor and releases EDRF/NO that spreads to vascular smooth muscle, causing an increase in guanosine $3'5'$-cyclic monophosphate (cGMP) with vasodilation.
- As secondary messengers, G proteins make the connection with the phosphatidylinositol pathway, which, in turn, mobilizes the intracellular calcium necessary for the formation of NO from L-arginine by the action of nitric oxide synthase (NOS).
- Among the blockers of the effects and synthesis of EDRF/NO, the most important are methylene blue (blockage at cGMP level); hemoglobin ("hijacker" or EDRF/NO scavenger); and the nitric (N^G-nitro-L-arginine, L-NOARG) and methylated (N^G-monomethyl-L-arginine, L-NMMA) forms of L-arginine which are NOS blockers.
- Endothelium produces at least four "families" of endothelium-derived contracting factors (EDCFs), in balance with the endothelial vasodilating factors. These contractile factors can be classified into EDCF 1s – factors dependent on the cyclooxygenase pathway; EDCF 2s – the family of endothelins that are vasoconstrictor polypeptides; EDCF 3s – vasoconstrictors released during hypoxia; and EDCF 4s – oxygen free radicals independent of the cyclooxygenase pathway.
- Some data evolving NO synthases are noteworthy. The so-called "constitutive" (cNOS) forms depend on Ca^{2+} and calmodulin and release. The "inducible" (iNOS) is regulated at a pre-transcriptional level and induced by cytokines.

References

1. Evora PR. The scientific impact of the nitric oxide discovery as vasodilator and endogenous antithrombotic agent. Arq Bras Cardiol. 1993;61(1):3–5.
2. Evora PRB, Pearson PJ, Schaff HV. Alguns aspectos da função endotelial em cirurgia cardíaca. Rev Bras Cir Cardiovasc. 1993;8(3):195–214.
3. Evora PRB, Pearson PJ, Discilgil B, Seccombe JF, Oeltjen M, Schaff H. Oxido nítrico e substância vasoativas derivadas do endotélio: papel no controle do tônus vascular. Revista da Sociedade de Cardiologia do Estado de São Paulo. 1996;6(2):129–37.
4. Weinbaum S, Zhang X, Han Y, Vink H, Cowin SC. Mechanotransduction and flow across the endothelial glycocalyx. Proc Natl Acad Sci U S A. 2003;100(13):7988–95.

5. Torres LN, Sondeen JL, Ji L, Dubick MA, Torres Filho I. Evaluation of resuscitation fluids on endothelial glycocalyx, venular blood flow, and coagulation function after hemorrhagic shock in rats. J Trauma Acute Care Surg. 2013;75(5):759–66.
6. Schott U, Solomon C, Fries D, Bentzer P. The endothelial glycocalyx and its disruption, protection and regeneration: a narrative review. Scand J Trauma Resusc Emerg Med. 2016;24:48.

Part II
Particularities of Endothelial Dysfunction in Different Types of Shock

Chapter 3
Circulatory Shock: A Conceptual and Practical Approach

The Best Definition of Circulatory Shock

Perhaps the best approach to defining cardiocirculatory shock is that of Robert Hardaway, who begins his discussion by stating, "what shock is not." This approach is interesting because it demonstrates the entire evolution of the circulatory shock concept as the pathophysiological concepts have changed. Thus, shock is not (1) caused by low blood pressure – due to the hypothalamic-pituitary-adrenal axis (catecholamines and cortisol release), normal and even supranormal blood pressure can be maintained; (2) pH does not necessarily accompany it – it can be normal or even alkalotic depending on the endogenous bicarbonate production and compensatory hyperventilation; (3) it is not always accompanied by low cardiac output – there are hyperdynamic states associated, for example, with sepsis; (4) it is not due to the exhaustion of the adrenal gland – in pre-death, catecholamines plasma levels are high; (5) arteriole dilation does not necessarily exist – the rule is that vasoconstriction occurs; and (6) there is not necessarily hypovolemia – an example is a cardiogenic shock resulting from acute myocardial infarction. After these considerations, it would remain to define "what shock is," and, in search of a universal definition, it was concluded that the best definition of the shock state would be "inadequate capillary perfusion" or, simply, "bad tissue perfusion" [1].

Cardiocirculatory Shock Classification

There are at least two classifications mostly used for shock: the "etiological" classification and the "pathophysiological" classification [2].

By etiological classification, shock can be classified as (1) hypovolemic due to bleeding, plasma loss (burns), and water and electrolytes loss (diarrhea, vomit, heat

P. R. Barbosa Evora et al., *Vasoplegic Endothelial Dysfunction*, https://doi.org/10.1007/978-3-030-74096-2_3

stroke); (2) cardiogenic due to acute myocardial infarction, pulmonary embolism, or cardiac tamponade; (3) septicemic due to infections; (4) neurogenic due to brain and spinal cord injuries, barbiturates, and spinal anesthesia; and (5) anaphylactic, from medication, insect bites, and iodinated contrasts (Table 3.1). This classification has some conceptual errors, for example, pulmonary embolism and cardiac tamponade as causes of cardiogenic shock. In reality, in these situations there is a ventricular filling insufficiency and not a myocardium insufficiency.

The "pathophysiological" classification is more interesting because it is associated with the shock mechanism: (1) hypovolemic – with the same characteristics as the previous classification; (2) cardiogenic – is practically related to an acute myocardial infarction; (3) obstructive – due to filling deficiency caused by pulmonary embolism or cardiac tamponade; and (4) distributive – where shocks that occur with vasoplegia (septicemic, anaphylactic, and neurogenic) are included (Table 3.2).

The Multisystem View and the Clinical Presentation of the Cardiocirculatory Shock

From a clinical point of view, it has been observed that due to the recent progress in assistance to medical emergencies, such as cardiocirculatory shock, patients who manage to survive may exhibit a syndrome. This was previously accepted as associated with severe infections and received several names: "multiple organ failure," "sequential system failure," "multisystem failure," and "multiorgan failure," among others. The cardiocirculatory shock causes this syndrome due to vital organ hypoxia. As mentioned, this is a consequence of medical care improvements since, in the past, patients had died early, often with isolated organic insufficiency, with no time to progress sequentially. Mortality related to the number of organs involved ranges from 23 to 30% for one insufficient organ, 44 to 60% for two, 79 to 85% for three, and 100% for four affected organs [2].

The consequences of a circulatory shock cause the functional impairment of vital organs that present predictable responses. These organs, when affected, are not very versatile in their manifestations [2].

The central nervous system presents cerebral edema and, eventually, seizures. Thus, mental fogging and agitation can be related to poor cerebral perfusion.

Table 3.1 Etiological classification of shock

Hypovolemic shock: major bleeding, plasma loss from burns, water, and electrolytes loss
Cardiogenic shock: acute myocardial infarction, cardiac arrhythmias, pulmonary embolism, cardiac tamponade
Septicemic shock: bacterial infections, fungal infections
Anaphylactic shock: drugs, food, insect bites, iodinated contrasts
Neurogenic shock: traumatic brain injuries, spinal anesthesia, barbiturates

Table 3.2 Pathophysiological classification of shock	*Hypovolemic shock:* major bleeding, plasma loss from burns, water, and electrolytes loss
	Cardiogenic shock: acute myocardial infarction
	Obstructive shock: pulmonary embolism and cardiac tamponade
	Distributive shock: septicemic shock, anaphylactic shock, and neurogenic shock

The lung responds with interstitial edema, which is the pathophysiological basis of the condition called adult respiratory distress syndrome (ARDS), with the advent of respiratory distress and unsaturation of the arterial blood. It often requires respiratory assistance with the need for intubation and the use of mechanical respirators.

The heart presents heart failure with dyspnea, edema, and cardiac arrhythmias.

Kidney hypoperfusion causes oliguric, or non-oliguric acute renal failure, which may lead to the need for dialysis.

The digestive tract responds with hemorrhages due to stress ulceration, in addition to cholecystitis. In addition, hepatocyte failure occurs with decreased glycogen stores and intractable hyperglycemia.

The musculoskeletal system may become insufficient due to the lesion catabolism.

The metabolism system can fail to meet the needs of the whole organism. Furthermore, due to tissue damage, thromboplastin penetrating the bloodstream ends up presenting disorders of disseminated intravascular coagulation. The reticuloendothelial system can produce antibodies with a higher possibility of secondary infection.

From acid-base and hydrolyzolytic balance, the most common disorders are hyperkalemia, hyponatremia, and metabolic acidosis compensated by respiratory alkalosis, which evolves into mixed acidosis with the worsening of the condition.

Finally, the tissue hypoxia phenomenon is universal, and the "multiple organ failure" syndrome defines the tragic consequences and sequelae of the shock state very well.

Multisystem Monitoring

Technological developments have led to an unbelievable sophistication in shock monitoring. The advent of this technology brought some frustration in terms of risk-benefit since it did not change the prognosis of conditions such as cardiogenic shock after acute myocardial infarction and the advanced sepsis associated with ARDS where proteins, overcoming the pulmonary interstitium, reach the alveoli [2].

Concerning the central nervous system, it is worth mentioning the Glasgow-Pittsburgh scale, which standardized the neurological examination and the intracranial pressure (ICP) measurement, which abolished empiricism in the cerebral edema treatment. Thus, osmotherapy and hyperventilation started to be used only in the condition of ICP greater than 20 mmHg and not as a routine.

Cardiac function monitoring includes, in addition to heart rate, measurement of heart rate and central venous pressure (CVP), the latter being discussed within the therapeutic principles. The excellent weapon for understanding specific pathophysiology and the treatment of shock was the advent of what was conventionally called hemodynamics at the bedside. This technology was made possible by the use of the Swan-Ganz catheter, which, in addition to measuring the pressures of right heart cavities, allows the measurement of cardiac output by thermodilution and the measurement of wedge pressure, which corresponds to the left atrial pressure. Thus, it became possible to monitor left ventricular function through a venous catheter.

Respiratory function monitoring is associated with the control of respiratory function (chest X-ray, respiratory volumes) and acid-base balance by interpreting arterial blood gases.

The digestive system is monitored, mainly, by the observation of hematemesis and/or melena (emphasizing the role of gastrointestinal endoscopy), jaundice, glycemia, liver, and pancreatic enzyme.

Renal function is assessed by observing diuresis and the measurements of nitrogenous compounds (urea and creatinine) and electrolytes.

Coagulation is assessed by coagulogram and by some signs with easy bleeding, ecchymosis, and petechiae. The immunological activity, intimately linked to the blood, is already possible to be monitored, among others, by the complement activity and immunoglobulin dosage.

Treatment of the Cardiocirculatory Shock

Treatment of the Cause Shock treatment should be aggressive and started early. The fundamental therapy objective is to treat the cause, correct the hemodynamic change, and, at the same time, neutralize abnormalities resulting from poor tissue perfusion [2].

Sequential Hemodynamic Reasoning One of the most sensible approaches to treating shock is the approach with data from cardiovascular physiology. Except for distributive shock that occurs with normal or high cardiac output, the cardiocirculatory shock implies low cardiac output. Thus, sequential reasoning based on the cardiac output formula provides subsidies in the circulatory shock treatment.

The cardiac output represents the product of stroke volume by heart rate, and stroke volume depends on the patient's blood volume and myocardial contractility, mainly left ventricular function. These are the elements to be considered, in a global and orderly way, in shock therapy: heart rate, blood volume, and myocardial contractility.

The heart rate, in general, is already increased by the reaction of the sympathetic nervous system. However, in exceptional situations, it can be low, and, since it is directly proportional to the cardiac output and its increase, it can be a therapeutic resource. Options for its improvement are vagal block by the use of atropine, beta-adrenergic stimulation by isoproterenol, or electrical stimulation by a cardiac pacemaker. It should be noted that the increase in heart rate should not exceed the limit of 120 bpm, above which there is impairment of the left coronary perfusion which occurs 75% in cardiac diastole.

Volume replacement, as mentioned earlier, is the cornerstone of shock treatment. Any other therapy should be taken after adequate volume restoration. Most failures in shock treatment are that this axiom is not adequately considered.

When the patient is tachycardic and with elevated CVP, consideration should be given to acting on the third determining factor of cardiac output, myocardial contractility. If the use of cardiocirculatory drugs does not improve the situation of low cardiac output, the relativity of the upper limits of the CVP measurement is considered, that is, it may be elevated due to right ventricular dysfunction, and the patient still needs an infusion of liquids. In the absence of pulmonary capillary pressure measurement with the Swan-Ganz catheter, the so-called overload test or fluid provocation test should be used, to be performed as follows: (a) Take note of the basic CVP. (b) Quickly infuse 200 mL of a colloid solution (today the most used and safe are starch-based solutions), and study the behavior of CVP. If it does not rise, the patient is not in danger of fluid overload, and more volume should be administered. In this condition, an apparently paradoxical response may occur with decreased CVP, meaning that the filling volume of the left ventricle was reduced despite high CVP. (c) If the CVP increases by 5 cmH$_2$O or more and falls to the initial levels after 10–15 minutes, the patient can still receive fluids with care. (d) If the CVP increases and does not fall later, the infusion rate should be reduced as the myocardial contractility component is undoubtedly the determinant of cardiocirculatory instability (Fig. 3.1).

Particularities of the Treatment of Hypovolemic Shock

Volume replacement should be concomitant with the control of blood, plasma, and water/electrolyte loss. For volume replacement, there are so-called colloid solutions (blood, plasma, albumin, Dextran, starch) and crystalloid solutions (saline, balanced electrolyte solutions, Ringer, Ringer-lactate). Colloids remain for 2–6 hours in the intravascular space, whereas crystalloids leave this space after 10–15 minutes, passing to the interstitial spaces. The volume replacement objective is to restore the extracellular space globally, that is, there must be simultaneous replacement of both the intravascular and the interstitial, to ensure the nutrition of the noble element that is the cell. Previously, the concept of volume replacement was that of "administration of similar liquids," that is, blood was only given to those who lost blood and plasma to those who lost plasma. With this conduct, many patients died with

Fig. 3.1 Sequential
hemodynamic reasoning

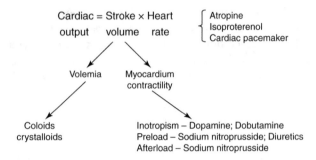

"unexplained metabolic acidosis," reported in the Second World War and the Korean War, even though they restored their blood volume. It is known today that the "unexplained acidosis" consisted of replacing only the intravascular (blood and/or plasma), without adequate nutrition of the cell due to the lack of replacement of the interstitial water space. Therefore, extracellular alternative implies the judicious use of both types of solutions and crystalloid colloid for the replacement of extracellular fluid (intravascular and interstitial). As a general rule, blood or plasma is used according to the hematocrit, which classically must be kept at around 30%, and crystalloids will be chosen according to their composition in electrolytes and the patient's ionogram. Among the so-called synthetic substitutes for plasma, gelatins are known to not act as colloids. The only synthetic colloid that has been accepted for a long time is Dextran, and its use is limited to the volume of 1000 mL, above which it can cause hemorrhagic disorders due to its antiplatelet activity. Both gelatins and dextrans have practically fallen out of use, with starch-based solutions being the most used today. In emergencies, therefore, and until blood or plasma is obtained, crystalloids should be used, which can restore the intravascular to a base of 3–4 times lost volume. It should be emphasized that its overuse, often uncontrollable, is the primary cause of interstitial pulmonary edema with respiratory failure (ARDS), a finding reported by the Americans in the Vietnam War [2].

Increasing evidence shows that aggressive strategies for resuscitation with crystalloids are associated with cardiac and pulmonary complications, gastrointestinal dysmotility, coagulation disorders, and immune and inflammatory disorders. Due to the large volumes of fluids administered, imbalances of intracellular and extracellular osmolarity may occur. Disturbances in cell volume can disrupt various regulatory mechanisms responsible for keeping the inflammatory cascade under control. Several authors have demonstrated the harmful effects of extensive crystalloid strategies based on resuscitation with large volumes of crystalloid, mainly pulmonary complications in specific populations submitted to surgical procedures. Also, a restrictive policy has been associated with a decrease in frequency and shorter recovery time from acute respiratory distress syndrome and tends to shorter hospital stays and lower mortality. Early hemorrhagic shock resuscitation, predominantly with saline, has been associated with cardiac dysfunction and lower cardiac output, as well as higher mortality.

Several researchers have evaluated the potential risk factors for the development of abdominal compartment syndrome and have universally observed the overuse of crystalloids as the primary determinant. This may be a return to the early 1970s and 1980s, when it was more sensible to restrict crystalloids to avoid interstitial edematous complications, especially from the respiratory system point of view.

Losses to the Third Space

Another point to be highlighted are the so-called losses to the third space, formed next to the interstitial. The losses to the third space must be replaced as if they were external losses. Once the shock is treated, after 36–72 hours, this phenomenon will begin to resolve with fluid return to the intravascular. At that moment, care should be taken to restrict venous replacement, and, if necessary, use diuretics and even resort to dialysis processes. Failure to perceive the internal redistribution of fluids may lead to heart and/or respiratory failure and the consequent death, despite all the effort and good initial success [2].

Particularities of Cardiogenic Shock Treatment

The performance on myocardial contractility should aim at its determinants: contractility itself, cardiac preload related to the complacency nervous territory, and afterload, associated with peripheral vascular resistance and increased afterload. Cardiotonics (dopamine, dobutamine, isoproterenol, digital, calcium) may be used to improve contractility and cardiac preload and, consequently, in decreasing the venous return and heart distension (making it work within the limits of the Frank-Starling law), venulodilators (morphine, nitrates, nitroglycerin, sodium nitroprusside, diuretics) are used. To decrease the afterload, thus facilitating the ejection of the stroke volume, arteriodilators (hydralazine, sodium nitroprusside, and alpha-blockers) are used. Based on these facts, the combination of dopamine and/or dobutamine with sodium nitroprusside is currently used routinely to act on the cardiogenic component of any type of shock.

The association of dopamine and/or dobutamine with sodium nitroprusside, considered as the best option for the clinical control of cardiogenic shock, is not enough to decrease mortality by 70–80%. For this reason, with particular advantage, there is the resource of mechanical circulatory assistance: intra-aortic balloon and artificial hearts. The oldest, practical, and most established method of mechanical circulatory support is diastolic aortic counterpulsation using the intra-aortic balloon [2].

Particularities of Distributive Shock Treatment

The distributive shock (septicemic, anaphylactic, and neurogenic) treatment involves the use of vasoconstrictors. The vasoconstrictor of choice is norepinephrine because it does not have a positive chronotropic effect (until it should decrease the heart rate) and acts as a coronary artery dilator. Adrenaline, noradrenaline, and metaraminol can be used in three situations: when there is an anaphylactic component, present neurogenic participation, and when hypotension persists, despite all therapeutic measures. The latter is an exception indication since, even to the detriment of peripheral perfusion and other vital organs, it is necessary to maintain "a pressure head" at the root of the aorta, to guarantee the heart and brain perfusions [2].

In the case of distributive shock, there is relative hypovolemia that must be handled with care since, in this type of shock, there is an increase in vascular permeability with excessive leakage of fluids into the "third space." It should be used, depending on the needs of hemodynamics, but never forgetting that the primary therapeutic weapon is the use of vasoconstrictors.

Multisystem Therapeutics

As the present text has sought to present multisystem conceptual aspects, it is interesting to adopt this approach to complement the general therapeutic aspects [2].

For the cerebral edema treatment, osmotherapy is used (the most used is mannitol), and corticoids (inflammatory processes and neoplasms). Hyperventilation is a resource widely used to control intracranial hypertension, as long as PCO_2 levels below 25 mmHg are not maintained, as hypocapnia is one of the most potent stimuli for cerebral vasoconstriction.

The respiratory failure treatment requires the support of mechanical respiratory assistance, physical therapy techniques for alveolar recruitment, and the use of positive end-expiratory pressure (PEEP). Also, the use of diuretics, bronchodilators, corticosteroids, and antibiotics are specific options.

Hemorrhages are almost entirely controlled by digestive endoscopy. For renal function, dialysis processes and the use of diuretics (furosemide) are the primary resources.

Concomitantly with the treatment of the shock state, the acid-base and hydroelectrolytic balance must be corrected.

Heparin is useful in patients with disseminated intravascular coagulation, at a dose of 1000–1500 units an hour, in a continuous venous infusion.

Antibiotics are administered, especially in septic shock, according to the clinical suspicion of the infection and, if possible, based on cultures for aerobic and anaerobic bacteria.

Corticosteroids use is the subject of considerable controversy. Their widespread use was based on experimental facts that demonstrate that they are positive inotropes, alpha-blockers, but what is expected of them is the stabilization of the lysosome membrane, preventing cell death by releasing its enzymes and, consequently, preventing the shock irreversibility. The most widely used corticosteroid is methylprednisolone because it is less mineralocorticoid and depresses the adrenal gland functionless when compared to other corticosteroids. Corticosteroid pulse therapy use was questioned in the late 1980s by the work published by Roger Bone in the United States. This author demonstrated, in a study involving a little less than 400 septic patients, that the methylprednisolone pulse was associated with a higher incidence of ARDS, less reversion of the condition of ARDS patients, and higher mortality on the fourteenth day of hospitalization. For these data, the use of corticoids in the treatment of shock is contraindicated. But if the immunosuppressive effect of the intravenous pulse is undesirable, there is no better option for the systemic inflammatory reaction, and the current consensus implies the use of corticosteroids in anti-inflammatory doses.

Other therapeutic options, such as the use of fibronectin and the use of immunoglobulins, anti-cytokine factors, unlike the experimental results, have never had clinical approval. The infusion of 10 units of cryoprecipitate (Factor VIII) would provide the patient's body with fibronectin, a protein capable of stimulating the opsonization reaction, with an increase in the body's immune response to sepsis. The use of naloxone, a powerful opioid antagonist, would act by inhibiting the release of brain beta-endorphins on hemodynamic changes in sepsis.

Concluding Remarks

- The best definition of the shock state would be "inadequate capillary perfusion" or, simply, "poor tissue perfusion."
- By the etiological classification, shock can be classified into (1) hypovolemic due to bleeding, plasma loss (burns), and water and electrolytes loss (diarrhea, vomit, heat stroke); (2) cardiogenic due to acute myocardial infarction, pulmonary embolism, or cardiac tamponade; (3) septicemic due to infections; (4) neurogenic due to brain and spinal cord injuries, barbiturates, and spinal anesthesia; and (5) anaphylactic due to medication, insect bites, and iodinated contrasts.
- The "pathophysiological" classification is more interesting because it is associated with the shock mechanism: (1) hypovolemic; (2) cardiogenic – associated with acute myocardial infarction; (3) obstructive due to filling deficiency caused by pulmonary embolism or cardiac tamponade; and (4) distributive due to vasoplegia (septicemic, anaphylactic, and neurogenic).
- Shock treatment must be aggressive and started early. The fundamental therapy objective is to treat the cause, correct the hemodynamic change, and, at the same time, neutralize abnormalities resulting from poor tissue perfusion.

- The volume replacement objective is to restore the extracellular space globally, that is, there must be simultaneous replacement of both the intravascular and the interstitial, to ensure the nutrition of the noble element that is the cell.
- In the case of distributive shock, there is a relative hypovolemia that must be handled with care since, in this type of shock, there is an increase in vascular permeability with excessive leakage of fluids to the "third space." Never forget that the main therapeutic weapon is the use of vasoconstrictors.

References

1. Hardaway RM. Wound shock: a history of its study and treatment by military surgeons. Mil Med. 2004;169(7):iv.
2. Evora PRB, Castro e Silva O. Circulatory shock, SIRS and endothelial dysfunction. A conceptual and practical approach. In: Paulo UoS, editor. 2017.

Chapter 4
Circulatory Shock, Ischemia-Reperfusion Injury, Systemic Inflammatory Response Syndrome (SIRS), and Multiple Organ Failure

Many factors associated with the cardiocirculatory shock (surgical trauma, ischemia-reperfusion of organs, changes in body temperature, and release of endotoxins) have been well documented as inducing a complex inflammatory response (SIRS). These factors include complement system activation, cytokines release, leukocytes activation, and adhesion molecule expression, in addition to the production of various substances such as oxygen free radicals, arachidonic acid metabolites, platelet activation factor (PAF), nitric oxide (NO), and endothelin (Fig. 4.1). This inflammatory cascade can contribute to the development of postoperative complications, including, but not limited to, respiratory failure, renal dysfunction, hemorrhagic disorders, neurological dysfunction, and changes in cardiac and liver function, vasoplegic endothelial dysfunction, and, ultimately, multiple organ failure [1].

The decision to include this chapter was based on the association of the concepts since they are always present when discussing vasoplegic endothelial dysfunction or vasoplegic syndrome. The pathophysiological link is the situation that involves distributive circulatory shock, a hyperdynamic state with low systemic vascular resistance, and arterial hypotension resistant to the effect of vasopressor amines.

Ischemia and Reperfusion Injury

The reperfusion injury is a term used to describe the functional and structural changes, which become apparent during the flow restoration after a period of ischemia. In addition to ischemia reversal, blood flow restoration can result in several deleterious effects like necrosis of irreversibly damaged cells, marked cell swelling, and nonuniform flow restoration for all portions of the tissue. This chaotic restoration of tissue flow is known as the no-reflow phenomenon, which is the result of a vicious circle of vascular endothelial dysfunction, reduced local perfusion, more dysfunctional changes, more edema, etc.

© The Author(s), under exclusive license to Springer Nature   29
Switzerland AG 2021
P. R. Barbosa Evora et al., *Vasoplegic Endothelial Dysfunction*,
https://doi.org/10.1007/978-3-030-74096-2_4

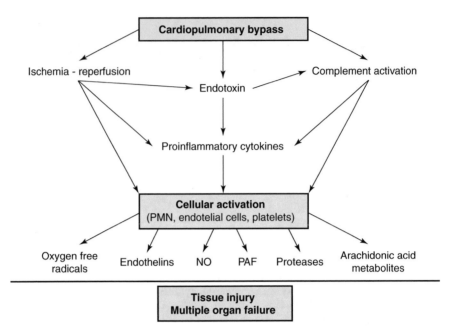

Fig. 4.1 Schematic representation of the inflammatory response generated by circulatory shock. PMN polymorphonuclear, NO nitric oxide, PAF platelet activation factor. (Adaptation by Wan et al. [1])

Metabolic disorders during ischemia or tissue hypoxia are very well established, but clinical and experimental evidence shows that the main events, which cause cellular and tissue dysfunction, are related to the subsequent reperfusion. When tissue blood flow is interrupted, many metabolic and enzymatic processes are affected. ATP reserves are rapidly depleted, there is an accumulation of lactate, the cell becomes acidic, and intracellular proteases are activated.

Also, increased capillary permeability causes tissue edema. Because the reversibility of this process is directly related to the duration of ischemia, the primary therapeutic objective is to restore reperfusion as quickly as possible. Although the benefit of early reperfusion is unquestionable, the reintroduction of oxygen in an ischemic environment initiates a complex chain of events leading to additional tissue damage and intracellular calcium accumulation.

Much has been studied in the last 40 years to define reperfusion injury pathogenesis. These studies include laboratory investigations, clinical observations, and extensive clinical trials. Current theories try to integrate three basic considerations: (1) the vascular relaxation impairment observed after ischemia-reperfusion injury, primarily endothelium-dependent vascular relaxations; (2) scavengers of oxygen free radicals limit reperfusion injury; and (3) blocking neutrophil activation and adhesion can reduce reperfusion injury.

As already clarified, reperfusion injury is a paradoxical and complex phenomenon of cell dysfunction exacerbation and increased cell death after blood flow restoration to previously ischemic tissues. It involves biochemical and cellular changes causing the production of oxidants and complement activation, which culminates in an inflammatory response, mediated by the interactions of neutrophil cells and platelets with the endothelium and between the cells themselves. The phenomenon has a local inflammatory reaction and systemic manifestations. Despite improvements in the image, intervention techniques, and pharmacological agents, reperfusion morbidity remains high.

Extensive research has favored the understanding of the various pathophysiological mechanisms involved and the development of potential therapeutic strategies. Preconditioning has emerged as a powerful method of easing myocardial ischemia-reperfusion and in transplant surgery. However, more research and well-designed trials are needed to bridge the gap between experimental evidence and clinical application.

Ischemic Preconditioning

Postconditioning can be defined as the process of limiting damage induced by ischemia-reperfusion injury by the repetitive application of short ischemic windows during early reperfusion. Zhao et al. (2003) were the first to describe this observation in dog hearts in 2003 and introduced the term postconditioning [2]. Staat et al. (2005) were the first to describe the clinical application in human hearts [3]. They described a 35% reduction in infarct size (as indicated by creatine kinase levels) in patients undergoing postconditioning. Although not prospective, at the time of the ischemic event, it is necessary to apply postconditioning within minutes for maximum benefit. Even a short delay of a few minutes can lead to a decrease in its effects. Yang et al. (2013) consider that a 10-minute delay after reperfusion dilutes the protection induced by preconditioning [4].

Remote Ischemia/Reperfusion Injury and Conditioning

A current concept tries to find a link between global ischemia followed by reperfusion, endothelial dysfunction, damage to organs remote to the organ(s) initially compromised, SIRS, and multiple organ failure. Hepatic ischemia, with subsequent reperfusion, is associated with secondary damage to organs located at a distance from the liver, with injuries attributed to oxidative stress mediators. However, other mediators such as arachidonic acid derivatives, metals, and NO may play some role [5].

The remote response causes leukocyte-dependent injury and free radicals' generation. The lesions can be mitigated by drugs such as allopurinol (xanthine oxidase inhibitor), N-acetyl-L-cysteine, mannitol (OH radical scavenger), and methylene blue (MB), suggesting that the NO generation, in addition to free radicals, may be involved in the injury. NO production in tissues located at a distance from the reperfused liver is not thoroughly studied. Thus, in general, there was substantial evidence of the pathophysiological role, in the multisystemic response to the cardiocirculatory shock, of (a) endothelial dysfunction/nitric oxide; (b) systemic inflammatory reaction, (c) lipid peroxidation (free radicals); and (d) leukocyte sequestration [5].

Remote Postconditioning

If the remote injury is a reality, the next step is logical thinking about the possibility of, as already mentioned, remote postconditioning. A strategy to prevent lethal reperfusion injury is to initiate, during reperfusion, transient ischemia, and reperfusion episodes in a tissue or an organ remote from the affected organ(s). This phenomenon is called remote ischemic postconditioning. Preliminary clinical trials are underway to determine whether transient upper and lower limb ischemia can reduce myocardial injury in patients with acute myocardial infarction. Recent experimental studies with rats demonstrated that a brief renal ischemia/reperfusion was able to protect the myocardium against lethal damage from reperfusion ischemia. However, the real therapeutic importance of remote postconditioning is still unknown [5].

Remote Preconditioning

Experimental studies have shown that the heart, liver, lung, intestine, brain, kidneys, and limbs are capable of producing remote preconditioning when subjected to brief ischemia/reperfusion. Intraconditioning between organs was first described in the heart, where brief ischemia in one territory led to protection in other areas.

Its clinical application has been demonstrated by the use of brief forearm ischemia in preconditioning the heart before myocardial revascularization and in reducing endothelial dysfunction of the contralateral limb. The protection of the heart has been demonstrated by the effects of remote preconditioning, obtained by brief ischemia of the lower limb, in children who underwent surgery with cardiopulmonary bypass for congenital heart disease treatments [5].

The stimulation of remote preconditioning presumably induces the release of biochemical messengers that act either through the bloodstream or via the neurogenic route, resulting in reduced oxidative stress and preservation of mitochondrial function. Studies have shown endothelial NO, free radicals, kinases, opioids, catecholamines, and KATP channels as the candidate mechanism for remote preconditioning. Experiments have shown suppression of pro-inflammatory genes, expression of antioxidant genes, and modulation of gene expression of remote ischemic preconditioning as a new method of preventing ischemia-reperfusion injury [5].

In conclusion, there is strong evidence to support remote ischemic preconditioning. The underlying mechanisms and signaling pathways should be clarified. Finally, the effective use of this type of preconditioning needs to be investigated in clinical settings.

Antioxidant Effect of Methylene Blue on Ischemia-Reperfusion Injury

Experiences from the 1990s, preceding the use of MB in the treatment of vasoplegic shock due to the main blocking action of guanylate cyclase, already supported the idea of how well its antioxidant activity would be useful in the injury of ischemia and reperfusion when administered in clinically concentrated concentrations before the molecular oxygen return [5].

The high affinity of MB for the iron-sulfuric nucleus of xanthine oxidase favors sequence I over sequence II, even in the presence of 100% O_2 during reoxygenation. In this sense, the role of MB as a "parasitic" electron receptor is defensible, diverting the electrons flow from the normal pathway within the enzyme to form blue leukomethylene at the level of the iron-sulfur centers. Although some studies suggest that univalently reduced MB is capable of reducing oxygen to superoxide, the rate of superoxide formation is relatively slow.

The result, the prevention of reactive oxygen species generation, is similar to the effect of superoxide dismutase (SOD). However, unlike SOD, MB having a low molecular weight and partly a fat-soluble agent is undoubtedly capable of penetrating cells and tissues because of its use as a rapidly penetrating histological dye. These properties can make MB an especially useful pharm for previously ischemic tissues [5].

Concluding Remarks

- Metabolic disorders during ischemia or tissue hypoxia are well established, but experimental and clinical evidence shows that the main events, which cause cellular and tissue dysfunctions, are related to the subsequent reperfusion.
- Preconditioning has emerged as a powerful method of mitigating myocardial ischemia-reperfusion and in transplant surgery. However, more research and well-designed trials are needed to bridge the gap between experimental evidence and clinical application.
- Postconditioning can be defined as the process of limiting damage induced by ischemia-reperfusion injury by repeated application of short ischemic windows during early reperfusion.

- Experiences from the 1990s, preceding the use of MB in the treatment of vaso-plegic shock by the main action of blocking guanylate cyclase, already supported the idea of how well its antioxidant action would be effective in the injury of ischemia and reperfusion when administered in clinically appropriate concentrations prior to the molecular oxygen return.

References

1. Wan S, LeClerc JL, Vincent JL. Inflammatory response to cardiopulmonary bypass: mechanisms involved and possible therapeutic strategies. Chest. 1997;112(3):676–92.
2. Zhao ZQ, Corvera JS, Halkos ME, Kerendi F, Wang NP, Guyton RA, et al. Inhibition of myocardial injury by ischemic postconditioning during reperfusion: comparison with ischemic preconditioning. Am J Physiol Heart Circ Physiol. 2003;285(2):H579–88.
3. Staat P, Rioufol G, Piot C, Cottin Y, Cung TT, L'Huillier I, et al. Postconditioning the human heart. Circulation. 2005;112(14):2143–8.
4. Yang S, Chou WP, Pei L. Effects of propofol on renal ischemia/reperfusion injury in rats. Exp Ther Med. 2013;6(5):1177–83.
5. Soares ROS, Losada DM, Jordani MC, Evora P, Castro ESO. Ischemia/reperfusion injury revisited: an overview of the latest pharmacological strategies. Int J Mol Sci. 2019;20(20):5034.

Chapter 5
Endothelial Dysfunction in Hemorrhagic Shock

Firstly, to reinforce the logic of this chapter, two studies chosen at random can be mentioned. Jeroukhimov et al. conducted a fascinating investigation to compare prehospital hypotensive resuscitation with volume resuscitation and find out whether reagents that inhibit the free oxygen radical formation, such as MB, can improve resuscitation and survival to treat hypovolemic states [1]. Ghiassi et al. conducted a study in dogs to assess prehospital resuscitation after refractory hemorrhagic shock with a combination of MB and lactated Ringer's limited volume solution [2].

Since the early 1990s, studies have investigated nitric oxide (NO) and the induction of calcium-independent nitric oxide synthase (NOS) in the development of vascular hyporeactivity to norepinephrine (NE) and vascular decompensation associated with hemorrhagic shock in experimental animals. Hypotheses were raised that this hyporeactivity would be mediated by the release of a NO boost by the constitutive NOS (eNOS), as it was reversed by N^G-nitro-L-arginine methyl ester (L-NMMA), a nonspecific iNOS/eNOS inhibitor, but has not been changed by dexamethasone, a selective iNOS inhibitor [3].

Vascular decompensation after prolonged periods of hemorrhagic shock was characterized by an inability of animals to maintain blood pressure, despite blood reinfusion. This progressive decrease in blood pressure is mediated by the advanced NO formation by iNOS, as it was prevented by L-NMMA or dexamethasone. A substantial increase in calcium-independent iNOS activity was observed in several organs after 150 and 330 minutes of hemorrhagic shock, being more pronounced in the lung, liver, and spleen. The hemorrhagic shock of 330 minutes, but not of 150 minutes, also caused hyporeactivity in rat aortic rings to vasoconstrictors, which was associated with the induction of iNOS activity in this tissue. Aortic hyporeactivity was prevented by pretreatment with dexamethasone in vivo and reversed by L-NMMA in vitro. Hemorrhagic shock was not associated with an increase in plasma endotoxin levels, showing that endotoxin does not count for iNOS induction in this model. Thus, excessive NO formation induces vascular hyporeactivity and decompensation in hemorrhagic shock, indicating that NOS inhibitors, particularly

P. R. Barbosa Evora et al., *Vasoplegic Endothelial Dysfunction*, https://doi.org/10.1007/978-3-030-74096-2_5

iNOS, could improve the therapeutic outcome of patients with hemorrhagic shock. Subsequently, human studies with NO synthesis inhibitors were associated with increased mortality and were abandoned for clinical use [3].

As in endotoxic shock, hemorrhagic shock leads to progressive vasodilation and reduced vascular responsiveness to the action of catecholamines. The onset of these vascular changes coincides and can play an essential role in the transition from the reversible phase to the irreversible step of shock. It is already well established that vascular hyporeactivity in hemorrhagic shock is not associated with changes in plasma levels of catecholamines or acidosis. However, until very recently it was believed that changes in vascular musculature, by themselves or with the participation of the neuroeffective junction effects, would be associated with vasoplegia.

Controlled bleeding in experimental animals leads to a progressive decrease in the pressure response to the action of vasoactive amines. It should be noted that this vascular hyporeactivity is not restored by retransfusion but can be reversed by pharmacological inhibition of NO synthesis. The early increased NO formation in the hemorrhage precedes the iNOS expression, suggesting the initial eNOS participation. It was demonstrated that the peroxynitrite formation also precedes the iNOS expression, suggesting an early formation by the reaction of the superoxide radical with the NO formed by the eNOS appearance. Prolonged periods of a hemorrhagic shock lead to iNOS expression. The mechanisms responsible for the iNOS induction in hemorrhagic shock are not well understood, and there are controversies regarding the roles of hypoxia and bacterial translocation. It should be noted that NOS inhibitors are harmful in the hemorrhagic shock treatment and that specific iNOS inhibitor, at least experimentally, may be useful in the treatment of progressive vascular failure in late states of hemorrhagic shock. Therefore, it can be suggested that NO could play a biphasic role, being cytoprotective during the early phase and cytotoxic in the late stage of hemorrhagic shock.

New Roles of Nitric Oxide in Hemorrhagic Shock

Recent developments in the field of hemorrhagic shock research regarding the NO review the pathogenesis of this condition. An analytical assessment focuses on the peroxynitrite actions, a reactive oxidant produced from the reaction of NO and superoxide. Another aspect is related to the new findings regarding the roles recently identified by the regulation of the inducible isoform of nitric oxide synthase (iNOS) in the expression of pro-inflammatory mediators in a state of hemorrhagic shock [3].

Although the severity and duration of the shock can dictate the time and extent of iNOS expression, it is now evident that the increased iNOS regulation can happen during hemorrhagic shock. Accumulated data indicate that iNOS expressed during shock contributes to vascular decompensation, as classically described by Wiggers [4]. Also, the presence of low iNOS levels at the time of resuscitation increases the inflammatory response that accompanies the reperfusion state. Drugs such as N6-(iminoetill)-L-lysine or genetic inactivation of iNOS (iNOS mice) that, inhibiting NOS, attenuates the activation of transcription factors such as nuclear factor kappa B (NFkappaB) and transcription transducer and activator 3 (STAT3) improve increases in interleukin-6 and levels of G-CSF messenger RNA in the lungs and liver. Also, the inhibition of iNOS could be a consequence of a marked reduction of the lung and liver damage produced by hemorrhagic shock. Thus, induced NO, in addition to being a "common final mediator" of hemorrhagic shock, is essential for increasing the inflammatory response in recovered hemorrhagic shock. Therefore, an evolutionary pathway that contributes to late tissue damage is configured, either directly through the formation of peroxynitrite, with its associated toxicities or, indirectly, through the amplification of the inflammatory response.

The Role of Peroxynitrite

Immunohistochemical and biochemical evidence demonstrate the production of peroxynitrite in a state of hemorrhagic shock. Peroxynitrite can initiate a wide range of toxic oxidative reactions. These reactions include initiation of tyrosine nitration, lipid peroxidation, direct inhibition of mitochondrial respiratory chain enzymes, inactivation of glyceraldehyde-3-phosphate dehydrogenase, inhibition of sodium/potassium ATPase membrane activity, inactivation of membrane sodium channels, and other oxidative proteins modifications. All these toxicities are likely to play a role in the hemorrhagic shock pathophysiology. A combined anti-inflammatory agent, mercapto-ethyl guanidine, which selectively inhibits peroxynitrite and iNOS, was able to prevent vascular failure and energy cell failure associated with late hemorrhagic shock. Peroxynitrite is a potent initiator of single-stranded DNA breakage, with subsequent activation of the nuclear poly enzyme (ADP ribose) synthetase (PARS), leading to the eventual severe depletion of cell energy, with possible evolution to necrosis or death. PARS-inhibiting drugs, such as 3-aminobenzamide or 5-iodine-6-amino-1,2-benzopyran, improve the hemodynamic status and prolong survival in rodent and pig models of severe hemorrhagic shock [5].

Endothelial Dysfunction Associated with the Use of Large Volumes of Crystalloid Solutions

Endothelial dysfunction is presumed to occur after hemorrhagic shock and resuscitation. This study uses an original large animal model to assess the effects of different resuscitation regimes on endothelial function. This is the first description of a large-scale animal model to assess EDRF/NO after hemorrhagic shock. Lactate Ringer (LR) requires resuscitation with volumes significantly larger than shed blood (SB) or LR followed by SB (SB). LR resuscitation leads to endothelial dysfunction, as determined by the decrease in endothelium-dependent relaxation (EDR), against

SB or LRSB. Resuscitation with blood products can preserve NO bioactivity when compared to crystalloid resuscitation in the adjustment of hemorrhagic shock [6].

Vasoactive Properties of Synthetic Plasma Substitutes

According to Poli-Figueiredo et al. (2006), there is a great need to develop a safe and efficient blood substitute to overcome the critical limitations of homologous blood transfusion. Currently, oxygen-carrying solutions based on hemoglobin-free cells with exchange properties similar to that of blood and with potential benefits over conventional transfusion are available, including abundant supplies, no transfusion reactions, no need for cross-testing, no risk for disease transmission, and long storage life. Several experimental studies have suggested that "hemoglobin-free" solutions are vasoactive agents. In animal models of hemorrhagic shock, small doses of these solutions were able to restore blood pressure, promote adequate tissue oxygenation, and improve survival, when compared to fluids without oxygen transport capacity. On the other hand, it has been shown that hemoglobin-induced vasoconstriction can result in decreased cardiac output, reduced blood flow to vital organs, and severe pulmonary hypertension. The "hemoglobin-free" solutions cause their pressure effects by binding and "sequestering" NO. Although hemoglobin inside red blood cells is the natural NO inactivator, when hemoglobin is free in solution, NO is inactivated to a greater extent. Finally, "hemoglobin-free" solutions are in an advanced stage of clinical testing; however, some concerns raised by experimental studies are not adequately considered for the clinical trial initiation [7].

The Possible Role of L-Arginine

Early administration of L-arginine (a NO precursor) may help to restore organ perfusion and reduce tissue damage after shock. This improvement in cardiovascular function was associated with the functional restoration of the immunodepressed cell, improving immune-mediated responses, with consequent attenuation of the massive inflammatory response found in such conditions [8].

Due to the decrease of neutrophil infiltrations, hemorrhage becomes more controllable by the L-arginine administration, with a reduction in liver damage. In addition, L-arginine treatment decreased the inflammatory response at the trauma site, improving the healing process after blood loss. Despite these promising results in animal models, none of the published clinical trials has shown L-arginine in doses higher than the standard of dietary practices on the outcome in critically ill patients.

Later, Wiggers (1942) created the classic model of fixed pressure hemorrhage. In this experiment, the animals were catheterized under anesthesia, allowing control of the blood volume removed and the desired hypotensive shock intensity [4]. The catheters also provided access to resuscitation and drug delivery. The main advantage of this model is that the degree and duration of hypotension are precisely controllable by monitoring blood pressure. These experiments showed that MB is safe in acute hypovolemic replacement and the beneficial effects on hemorrhagic shock are demonstrated only in association with volume replacement as soon as possible.

Concluding Remarks

- Jeroukhimov et al. conducted a fascinating investigation to compare prehospital hypotensive resuscitation with volume resuscitation and find out whether reagents that inhibit the formation of free oxygen radicals, such as MB, can improve resuscitation and survival to treat hypovolemic states.
- Ghiassi et al. carried out a study in dogs to evaluate prehospital resuscitation after refractory hemorrhagic shock with a combination of MB and Ringer's limited volume solution with lactate.
- Vascular decompensation after prolonged periods of hemorrhagic shock was characterized by an inability of animals to maintain blood pressure, despite blood reinfusion. This progressive decline in blood pressure is mediated by the advanced NO formation by iNOS because it was prevented by L-NMMA or by dexamethasone.
- As in endotoxic shock, hemorrhagic shock leads to progressive vasodilation and reduced vascular responsiveness to the action of catecholamines.
- Controlled bleeding in experimental animals leads to a progressive decrease in the pressure response to the action of vasoactive amines. It is emphasized that this vascular hyporeactivity is not restored by retransfusion but can be reversed by the pharmacological inhibition of NO synthesis.
- Although the severity and duration of the shock can dictate the time and extent of iNOS expression, it is now evident that the increased iNOS regulation can happen during hemorrhagic shock.
- LR resuscitation leads to endothelial dysfunction, as determined by the NO decrease in SB or LRSB transfusions. Resuscitation with blood-derived products can preserve the NO bioactivity compared to chronic resuscitation in the hemorrhagic shock adjustment.

References

1. Jeroukhimov I, Weinbroum A, Ben-Avraham R, Abu-Abid S, Michowitz M, Kluger Y. Effect of methylene blue on resuscitation after haemorrhagic shock. Eur J Surg Acta chirurgica. 2001;167(10):742–7.
2. Ghiassi S, Sun YS, Kim VB, Scott CM, Nifong LW, Rotondo MF, et al. Methylene blue enhancement of resuscitation after refractory hemorrhagic shock. J Trauma. 2004;57(3):515–21.

3. Kilbourn RG, Traber DL, Szabo C. Nitric oxide and shock. Disease-a-month: DM. 1997;43(5):277–348.
4. Wiggers CJ. The present status of the shock problem. Physiol Rev. 1942;22(1):74–123.
5. Szabo C, Modis K. Pathophysiological roles of peroxynitrite in circulatory shock. Shock. 2010;34 Suppl 1:4–14.
6. Savage SA, Fitzpatrick CM, Kashyap VS, Clouse WD, Kerby JD. Endothelial dysfunction after lactated Ringer's solution resuscitation for hemorrhagic shock. J Trauma. 2005;59(2):284–90.
7. Poli-de-Figueiredo LF, Cruz RJ Jr, Sannomiya P, Rocha ESM. Mechanisms of action of hypertonic saline resuscitation in severe sepsis and septic shock. Endocr Metab Immune Disord Drug Targets. 2006;6(2):201–6.
8. Loehe F, Bruns CJ, Nitsch SM, Angele MK. The role of L-arginine following trauma and blood loss. Curr Opin Clin Nutr Metab Care. 2007;10(1):80–7.

Chapter 6
Endothelial Dysfunction in Cardiogenic Shock

A clinical update written by Hochman (2003) targeted his thoughts on "expanding the paradigm" of cardiogenic shock as an acute myocardial infarction (AMI) complication [1].

A systemic inflammatory response (SIRS), complement activation, inflammatory cytokines release, inducible nitric oxide synthase (iNOS) expression, and vasodilation can now solely play a crucial position not only in the shock genesis but also on its evolution (Fig. 6.1).

New pathophysiological interpretations and treatments based totally on vasoplegia triggered through increased iNOS expression have been suggested, such as that

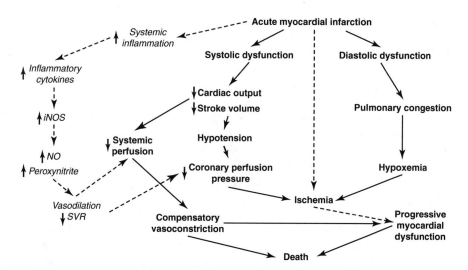

Fig. 6.1 Cardiogenic shock related with vasoplegia – Hochman's adaptation. (Adaptation from Hochman [1]). iNOS inducible nitric oxide synthase, NO nitric oxide, SVR systemic vascular resistance

© The Author(s), under exclusive license to Springer Nature
Switzerland AG 2021
P. R. Barbosa Evora et al., *Vasoplegic Endothelial Dysfunction*,
https://doi.org/10.1007/978-3-030-74096-2_6

used in human patients by Cotter et al. (2000), who administered nonspecific nitric oxide synthase (NOS) inhibitors N^G-monomethyl-L-arginine (L-NMMA) in 11 patients and N^G-nitro-L-arginine in a small randomized trial of 30 patients [2].

Cardiogenic shock, a devastating final result of acute myocardial infarction, is related to extraordinarily excessive mortality. Treatment techniques ought to center attention on rapid reperfusion and hemodynamic support. The first approach for new therapy is angiography and coronary revascularization by percutaneous intervention or myocardial revascularization surgery, with diastolic counterpulsation with an intra-aortic balloon pump [3].

Adjuvant pharmacological therapy is related to various agents, especially inotropic and vasopressors, which are additionally useful for hemodynamic support. However, these agents have shown no survival benefit, and their use is frequently based on clinical experience.

Experimental and clinical evidences suggest that a systemic inflammatory response, including iNOS upregulation, complement activation, and an inflammatory cytokines cascade, has a proven role in the improvement of cardiogenic shock. Moreover, new therapeutic strategies, including C5 inhibitors and NOS inhibitors, are being mixed with reasonable procedures, such as inotropic, vasopressor circulatory assistance, for the cardiogenic shock treatment.

Tilarginine is monomethyl L-N-arginine (L-NMMA) or N (G)-monomethyl-L-arginine HCL (L-NMMA), a nonselective NOS inhibitor, which has been studied in the cure of septic shock and cardiogenic shock complicating myocardial infarction. Despite the robust evidence that immoderate nitric oxide (NO) manufacturing plays an essential position in the septic shock pathogenesis, there is proof that this immoderate manufacturing might contribute to the cardiogenic shock pathogenesis after myocardial infarction. However, research on the consequences of NOS inhibition in these two problems have proved disappointing.

Therapy with L-NMMA used to be related to an excess mortality, in particular at doses of 5 mg/(Kg h), emphasizing that in septic and cardiogenic shocks, the consequences of a decrease remedy (1 mg/(Kg h)) were neutral. The excess mortality in patients with septic shock was nearly indeed the result of unfavorable hemodynamic changes caused with the aid of L-NMMA (decreased cardiac output, improved pulmonary vascular resistance, and reduced tissue oxygen supply).

The lack of activity in the nonspecific NO synthesis blockage in patients with cardiogenic shock after myocardial infarction may additionally have been due to the fact that the dose of L-NMMA was too low. Additional research using higher doses of L-NMMA (5 mg/(Kg h)) in conjunction with an inotropic guide could produce more recommended results. On the other hand, the use of an inducible NOS (iNOS) inhibition to reduce the pathological consequences of excessive NO production, leaving the beneficial impact of vascular NO production by endothelial eNOS, could prove to be of value. Animal studies and small trials with humans have proven to be encouraging, but a large study in humans (TRIUMPH), proposed to evaluate tilarginine (N^G-monomethyl-L-arginine, L-NMMA), was recently closed due to lack of effectiveness and trend towards increased mortality. This research assessed compounds with low selectivity for iNOS, and their failure may additionally have been due, in part, to the inhibition of other NOS isoforms, reinforcing the concept of future trials with other selective iNOS inhibitors [4].

The unfavorable evidence for the iNOS inhibition in cardiogenic shock led to an exceptional severe doubt: The tragedy of TRIUMPH for nitric oxide synthesis inhibition: where will we go from here? Methylene blue (MB) has been recognized as a guanylate cyclase inhibitor capable of abolishing vascular smooth muscle relaxation based on guanosine 3′5′-cyclic monophosphate (cGMP), without interfering with NO synthesis and without producing tissue necrosis associated with the use of NOS inhibitors. Thus, MB for all that has been written in this book could be a therapeutic option, not yet tested, for vasoplegia related to cardiogenic shock [5].

Concluding Remarks

- A systemic inflammatory response (SIRS), complement activation, inflammatory cytokines release, iNOS expression, and vasodilation can now solely play a crucial position not only in the shock genesis but also on its evolution.
- These pathophysiological aspects "expanded the paradigm" of cardiogenic shock complicating acute myocardial infarction, suggesting new interpretations and therapies.
- Evidence suggests that a systemic inflammatory response, including iNOS upregulation, complement activation, and a cascade of inflammatory cytokines, has a proven role in the improvement of cardiogenic shock.
- New therapeutic strategies, including C5 inhibitors and NOS inhibitors, are being mixed with reasonable procedures, such as inotropic, vasopressor circulatory assistance, for the cardiogenic shock treatment.
- The unfavorable evidence for the iNOS inhibition in cardiogenic shock led to an exceptional severe doubt: The tragedy of TRIUMPH for nitric oxide synthesis inhibition: where will we go from here?
- Methylene blue (MB) has been recognized as a guanylate cyclase inhibitor capable of abolishing vascular smooth muscle relaxation based on guanosine 3′5′-cyclic monophosphate (cGMP), without interfering with NO synthesis and without producing tissue necrosis associated with the use of NOS inhibitors. Should it be a therapeutic option to be tested?

References

1. Hochman JS. Cardiogenic shock complicating acute myocardial infarction: expanding the paradigm. Circulation. 2003;107(24):2998–3002.
2. Cotter G, Kaluski E, Blatt A, Milovanov O, Moshkovitz Y, Zaidenstein R, et al. L-NMMA (a nitric oxide synthase inhibitor) is effective in the treatment of cardiogenic shock. Circulation. 2000;101(12):1358–61.

3. Reynolds HR, Hochman JS. Cardiogenic shock: current concepts and improving outcomes. Circulation. 2008;117(5):686–97.
4. Howes LG, Brillante DG. Expert opinion on tilarginine in the treatment of shock. Expert Opin Investig Drugs. 2008;17(10):1573–80.
5. Bailey A, Pope TW, Moore SA, Campbell CL. The tragedy of TRIUMPH for nitric oxide synthesis inhibition in cardiogenic shock: where do we go from here? Am J Cardiovasc Drugs. 2007;7(5):337–45.

Chapter 7
Endothelial Dysfunction in Distributive Shock

Since the 1990s, nitric oxide (NO) has been associated with vasoplegia of septic shock resistant to high doses of catecholamines. After exposure to bacterial endotoxin or specific cytokines, the inducible nitric oxide synthase (iNOS) expression occurs in a wide variety of tissues. This enzyme produces large NO amounts over long periods, closely related to the pathophysiological changes in sepsis. In some cells, including macrophages, NO synthesized by iNOS is toxic and appears to be an essential mediator in the defense of the host. Animal and in vitro studies have shown that this NO release into other tissues can cause extreme vasodilation, damage to the cell population and heart failure [1].

NO synthesis inhibitors can reverse hypotension caused by endotoxin and cytokine, and these agents could, in theory, constitute a modern therapeutic approach to severe septic shock. Preliminary studies in humans suggest that NOS inhibition improves blood pressure and stabilizes hemodynamics, but mortality rates remain undetermined. It can be said that the use of synthesis inhibitors was associated with increased mortality compared to the control group in humans, causing multicenter studies to be interrupted. The participation of the overproduction of NO by the iNOS expression is evident, leading to a vasoplegia state that is irresponsible to high doses of catecholamines [2].

Contrary to these concepts, which are already established for septicemic shock, there is little experimental evidence that relates to increasing NO production as a pathophysiological factor in anaphylactic shock, whose secondary mediators are different. Systemic anaphylaxis is associated with the acute release of substances such as histamine, leukotrienes, and platelet activation factor, although there is experimental evidence that there is no increase in pro-inflammatory cytokines. It is not surprising that the marked iNOS expression is not found in systemic

P. R. Barbosa Evora et al., *Vasoplegic Endothelial Dysfunction*, https://doi.org/10.1007/978-3-030-74096-2_7

anaphylaxis. On the other hand, there is an increase in NO production due to eNOS expression, which can be associated with early vascular hyporeactivity, with acute hypotension, observed in anaphylactic shock [2].

The use of NOS inhibitors in the experimental treatment of anaphylactic shock is questionable. NOS inhibition can increase blood pressure, but with a significant decrease in cardiac output. Also, the NO produced by the bronchial epithelium plays an essential role in counterbalancing anaphylactic bronchoconstriction, and the use of NOS inhibitors could worsen this clinical condition. These concepts, taken together, seem to show that NOS inhibitors have a limited role in anaphylactic shock treatment. This makes room for another therapeutic modality that does not interfere with NOS production, but rather with its effect on vascular smooth muscle, justifying guanylate cyclase inhibition, preventing the increase of guanosine $3'5'$-cyclic monophosphate (cGMP) that is responsible for vasodilation. Thus, methylene blue (MB) gains space to be tested in this type of circulatory shock [1].

Regarding neurogenic shock, studies on the participation of NO in vasoplegia are associated with it, and very few reviews are found in the specialized literature.

Inhibition of Nitric Oxide Synthesis as a Therapeutic Proposal for Vasoplegia Associated with Shock

When sepsis occurs, the first change in the circulatory system is the hypotension resulting from the dilation of systemic blood vessels. Although the NO and NOS relationship during sepsis is not well understood, it is believed that cytokines cause refractory hypotension and failure of the circulatory system due to LPS originating from bacteria. Subsequently, large NO volumes are produced.

NOS inhibition in sepsis can lead to liver and intestinal damage, increased platelet aggregation, pulmonary vasoconstriction, and expanded and reduced cardiac output. Also, the cellular biochemistry defense against exogenous pathogens could be impaired by the NOS inhibition. NOS inhibitors can have long-lasting effects that are not always predictable, limiting their use in a clinical setting. NOS inhibition to restore hypotension is still connected with many uncertainties and evident adverse side effects.

More knowledge about the NO role in septicemic shock and the participation of different NOS, which can be selectively inhibited, is needed. It should be noted that studies in humans had to be interrupted after the observation of a significant increase in mortality due to the use of NO synthesis inhibitors.

The Inhibition of Guanylate Cyclase by Methylene Blue as a Therapeutic Proposal for Vasoplegia Associated with Shock

Because of all the concepts discussed, MB seems to be the most reasonable therapeutic proposal since it does not interfere with NO synthesis and because it is a medication widely used in other clinical conditions. MB action implies guanylate cyclase inhibition, preventing the cGMP elevation and, consequently, avoiding NO-mediated endothelium relaxation (Fig. 7.1) [1].

The use of MB in patients with septic shock, in the infusion of $1–2$ mg.Kg^{-1}, is already established, providing an increase in blood pressure by inhibiting the NO action in vascular smooth muscle.

The NO release has been implicated in the cardiovascular septicemic shock changes. Since guanylate cyclase is the endothelium-dependent relaxation enzyme, MB is a potent inhibitor of this enzyme and an essential option for the sepsis vasoplegia treatment. A study in humans showed that MB increased the mean arterial pressure (MAP) and stroke volume in septicemic and shocked patients. The other parameters, obtained through the hemodynamic research at the bedside, did not show significant changes, and in some of the studied patients, the effect was not sustained, and, for this reason, a new dose was administered in an intravenous bolus

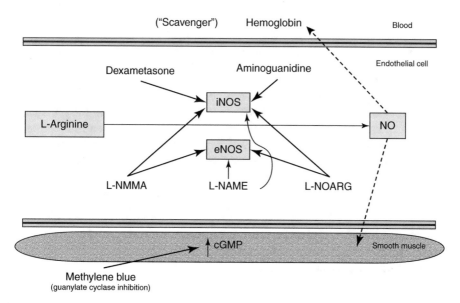

Fig. 7.1 Nitric oxide blockers, highlighting that hemoglobin and methylene blue are independent blockers of synthesis from L-arginine. NO nitric oxide, cGMP guanosine 3′5′-cyclic monophosphate, eNOS endothelial nitric oxide synthase, iNOS inducible nitric oxide synthase, L-NMMA N^G-monomethyl-L-arginine, L-NAME N^G-nitro-L-arginine methyl ester, L-NOARG N^G-nitro-L-arginine

of 2 mg.Kg^{-1} of the MB, observing the same initial effects. No adverse side effects were observed regarding the failure to sustain that the initial impact led to the adoption of MB's continuous infusion after the initial intravenous bolus.

In a bibliographic search, as wide as possible, the use of MB in the clinic to treat anaphylactic shock is found only in the works of Evora et al. [2].

The excellent results obtained in 13 clinical cases suggest the fundamental role of NO in the anaphylactic shock pathophysiology, raising MB to a condition of choice, or even priority, in its therapy. The accumulation of clinical experience may confirm these impressions. The MB dosages used (3.0 mg.Kg^{-1}) were adopted based on the knowledge acquired in the sepsis vasoplegia treatment and the methemoglobinemia treatment. This dose is safe since the lethal dose of MB, determined experimentally in goats, is 40 mg.Kg^{-1} [2].

Vasopressin-Dependent Mechanisms

Landry et al. (1997) have shown that vasopressin levels in septic shock are abnormally low [3]. This fact supports the hypothesis that in sepsis there may be a decrease in vasopressin stocks or a baroreflex dysfunction, causing insufficient vasopressin secretion. These authors also reported sepsis situations with refractory hypotension, which was recovered by the injection of vasopressin, which led to a decrease in catecholamine requirements.

Considering the similarities of the inflammatory response in sepsis and vasoplegia after cardiopulmonary bypass (CPB), Argenziano et al. (1997) published a retrospective analysis of 40 cases of distributive shock after cardiac surgery, treated with vasopressin [4].

These same authors included their experience with this drug, heart transplantation, and patients undergoing mechanical circulatory assistance. In these patients, there was no hypertensive rebound, peripheral, or mesenteric ischemia, along with an improvement in blood pressure levels and a decrease in catecholamine needs. The efficiency and safety of this new and promising pressure agent need further observation.

Therapeutic Principles for the Treatment of Vasoplegic Endothelial Dysfunction Associated with Cardiocirculatory Shock

The first, and most important, concept concerns the restrictions on the use of non-specific inhibitors of NO synthesis (L-NMMA, LAME, etc.). Some points can be highlighted:

Corticosteroids are used to inhibit the inflammatory reaction and block the iNOS action.

Norepinephrine is used, as it is an amine that does not promote an increase in heart rate and may even decrease it.

MB is used (2 mg.Kg^{-1} of weight in intravenous "bolus" or half of the dose in "bolus," followed by the continuous infusion of additional dosages).

Injectable metoprolol is used (5 mg) to reverse the downregulation situation of beta receptors, which is a consequence of tachycardia and the use of amines.

Because of this phenomenon, fewer beta receptors are available for effective action of beta-adrenergic drugs, with tachyphylaxis occurring.

It is imperative to avoid excess volume replacement, and the main objective is to reverse vasoplegia with vasoconstrictors and MB. As hypotension is refractory to the use of amines, the use of MB has been lifesaving. Using vasopressin arginine is quite attractive, but there is still no clinical experience with this drug, although we have performed some experimental trials.

The NO action depends on the activation of the cGMP system. But, in addition to this mechanism of significant importance, we have also turned our attention to the adenosine 3'5'-cyclic monophosphate (cAMP) system, which is why we are using, almost as a routine, injectable beta-blockers (metoprolol), when the patient is very tachycardic. Another logical approach would be to inhibit NO synthesis with the use of specific inhibitors such as L-NAME and L-NMMA. However, this approach is open to criticism, involves ethical problems related to the use of new therapies, and blocks not only iNOS but also the physiological form of this enzyme (cNOS). The use of specific iNOS inhibition, for example, with aminoguanidine, remains in the logical and speculative territories.

Possible Paradigm Shift

The combination of three concepts should be useful for better results against the high mortality rates in critically ill patients. These three concepts are (1) "wide-spectrum vasopressors," (2) vasopressor economy strategies, and (3) protection against microcirculation. We believe that a combination of these three concepts will be useful to obtain better results against the high mortality rates in critically ill patients. Some observations should be mentioned based on these concepts [5–8]. (4) "Broad-spectrum vasopressors" – this approach suggests that shock treatment should be started with the association of vasopressors with a different mechanism of action. Norepinephrine is used worldwide as a first-line vasopressor, but most often, it is routinely associated with catecholamines that target the same adrenergic receptors. However, it would be more logical to associate with a non-adrenergic vasopressor (vasopressin, angiotensin II). In other words, there is no sense in the association of noradrenaline with epinephrine. It should be emphasized that this view considers only receptor-dependent effects.

"Reserve strategies to support catecholamine vasopressors" have the same objective of protecting the microcirculation. Since fluids and amines are indisputable to maintain sufficient cardiovascular pressures for organ perfusion, inevitably, microcirculatory damage occurs over time. Therefore, it is mandatory to seek adjuvant therapeutic options to reduce the need for vasoactive support without compromising blood pressure [5, 6].

"Microcirculatory protection" is the oldest concept, assuming that even with blood pressure under control with increasing concentrations of amines, the failure in the microvasculature is inexorable. Therefore, special attention focused individually on microcirculation is correctly understood [9]. Cardiogenic shock may be associated with an inflammatory reaction. This possibility has motivated us experimentally and clinically in the use of MB in the last 25 years. Since the main targets of vasopressors are membrane receptors, wouldn't it be more logical to associate them with drugs that interfere with messengers beyond membranes?

Concluding Remarks

- After exposure to bacterial endotoxin or specific cytokines, the expression of inducible nitric oxide synthase (iNOS) occurs in a wide variety of tissues. This enzyme produces large NO amounts over long periods, closely related to the pathophysiological changes in sepsis.
- The participation of overproduction of nitric oxide (NO) by the expression of iNOS is evident, leading to a vasoplegia state irresponsible to high catecholamine doses.
- More knowledge about the NO role in septic shock and the participation of different synthases of nitric oxide, which can be selectively inhibited, is necessary. It should be noted that studies in humans had to be interrupted by the observation of a remarkable increase in mortality due to the use of NO synthesis inhibitors.
- Since guanylate cyclase is the endothelium-dependent relaxation enzyme, MB is a potent inhibitor of this enzyme and an essential option for the vasoplegia in sepsis treatment.

References

1. Petros A, Lamb G, Leone A, Moncada S, Bennett D, Vallance P. Effects of a nitric oxide synthase inhibitor in humans with septic shock. Cardiovasc Res. 1994;28(1):34–9.
2. Evora PR, Simon MR. Role of nitric oxide production in anaphylaxis and its relevance for the treatment of anaphylactic hypotension with methylene blue. Ann Allergy Asthma Immunol. 2007;99(4):306–13.
3. Landry DW, Levin HR, Gallant EM, Ashton RC Jr, Seo S, D'Alessandro D, et al. Vasopressin deficiency contributes to the vasodilation of septic shock. Circulation. 1997;95(5):1122–5.

4. Argenziano M, Choudhri AF, Oz MC, Rose EA, Smith CR, Landry DW. A prospective randomized trial of arginine vasopressin in the treatment of vasodilatory shock after left ventricular assist device placement. Circulation. 1997;96(9 Suppl):II-286–90.
5. Evora PRB. Broad spectrum vasopressors support sparing strategies in vasodilatory shock beyond the vascular receptors. Chest. 2020;157(2):471–2.
6. Evora PRB, Braile DM. "Vasopressor support sparing strategies": a concept to be incorporated as a paradigm in the treatment of vasodilatory shock. Braz J Cardiovasc Surg. 2019;34(1):I–II.
7. Squara P, Hollenberg S, Payen D. Reconsidering vasopressors for cardiogenic shock: everything should be made as simple as possible, but not simpler. Chest. 2019;156(2):392–401.
8. Chawla LS, Ostermann M, Forni L, Tidmarsh GF. Broad spectrum vasopressors: a new approach to the initial management of septic shock? Crit Care. 2019;23(1):124.
9. Nantais J, Dumbarton TC, Farah N, Maxan A, Zhou J, Minor S, et al. Impact of methylene blue in addition to norepinephrine on the intestinal microcirculation in experimental septic shock. Clin Hemorheol Microcirc. 2014;58(1):97–105.

Part III
Methylene Blue

Chapter 8
Methylene Blue

Chemical Characteristic

Methylene blue (MB) is presented as a dark blue-green crystalline powder that is odorless, soluble in water, alcohol, and chloroform, with a solubility constant in the water of 35.5 g.l^{-1}. It has a molecular weight of 319 g.mol^{-1}, and the 1% aqueous solution has a pH of 3. The powder is stable in sunlight and at a temperature of 15–25°C. It is important to note that the preparation containing zinc and the presentation in tetramethylthionine are not suitable for clinical use [1].

Pharmacokinetics

At gastric pH, MB is fully ionized. Oral absorption varies from 53% to 97%, achieving a peak in plasma after 30–60 minutes. The distribution volume is approximately 20 ml.kg^{-1}. Oral or intravenous administration has multi-compartmental pharmacokinetics with a terminal plasma half-life of 5–6 hours. MB is reduced in red blood cells and peripheral tissues in its primary metabolite (65–85%), leukomethylene. The metabolites are excreted mainly in the urine but also bile and feces. The non-metabolized fraction is excreted predominantly in the urine, causing a bluish-green discoloration [1].

Effect of Methylene Blue on sGC and NOS

The clinical history of MB dates to 1876. Paul Ehrlich, in 1910, used MB to distinguish living cells, which became blue, from dead cells that maintained their color. This line of research, in which Ehrlich tried to "attack bad cells and preserve good cells," gave this scientist the title of father of chemotherapy, noting that this German scientist was notable, among other things, for using MB in the treatment of malaria [1].

MB has been used in clinical practice for many years, for example, in the therapy of methemoglobinemia and as a urinary antiseptic, with no contraindications, to date, regarding its safe use. Thus, its use does not mean the introduction of a new drug that implies scientific and ethical rigors. The toxic and therapeutic effects of MB are due to the interaction with the nitric oxide/cyclic guanosine 3'5'-cyclic monophosphate pathway (NO/cGMP). MB blocks the inhibition of guanylate cyclase, closing the final effector pathway for NO release with vasodilating action. In addition to the impact on guanylate cyclase, it additionally inhibits NO synthesis by acting immediately on the heme group of endothelial nitric oxide synthase (eNOS) and inducible nitric oxide synthase (iNOS) [1].

MB inhibits sGC by binding to the heme group of this enzyme and inhibits NOS by oxidizing the Fe^{+2} molecule. It is suggested that MB is a more specific and potent NOS inhibitor since NO donor compounds are still capable of activating, even if partially, cGMP. Also, in the culture of endothelial cells, there is a report that MB inhibits the stimulation of guanylate cyclase even in the presence of nitrovasodilators. There are no data on the relative inhibition of NOS isoforms by MB nor on regional variations in eNOS inhibition. Thus, the indiscriminate NO/cGMP pathway inhibition will have an effect on the basal NO release in the microcirculation in a variable way, as well as the NO-mediated prostacyclin release, which can contribute to the different manifestations when inhibiting NO as an adjuvant therapy in vasoplegic syndrome and septicemia [1].

Methylene Blue and Coagulation

MB can be reduced in platelet aggregation for its consequences in the NO/cGMP pathway. Reduced platelet aggregation has been confirmed using experimental models of animals with damaged epithelium in the presence of MB [1].

The NO effects on platelet function are mediated by the inhibition of calcium-stimulated events: platelet activation, endothelial platelet adhesion, and platelet aggregation. These consequences happen in synergy with platelet thromboxane A2 (TXA2) and endothelial prostacyclin I2 (PGI-2). PGI-2 also exerts its effects on guanylate cyclase (sGC). However, it is coupled to adenosine 3'5'-cyclic monophosphate (cAMP) in each endothelial cell and platelets. The endothelial antiplatelet properties mediated via basal NO production are linked to the cGMP signaling pathway and the release of PGI-2 by cyclooxygenase (COX). The role of NO and PGI-2 is still controversial. Some believe that NO has a more significant effect on microcirculation and COX stimulation; others consider PGI-2 to be of great importance in the vasodilation of large-caliber vessels. Especially during pregnancy, the NO/PGI-2 system is extremely active and is involved in maintaining the blood supply to the placenta and fetus. Thus, manipulation of NO production and signaling can result in less vasodilation and higher platelet aggregation due to the involvement of direct and indirect effects caused by the decrease in NO and the production of PGI-2 mediated by NO. However, it is not yet known how the MB administered at some stage in cardiopulmonary bypass would affect the balance between anticoagulation and thrombosis [1].

In some reviews and laboratory studies, it was suggested the use of MB to reverse the action of heparin after cardiac surgery with the use of cardiopulmonary bypass (CPB). Attempts to reproduce such reviews in laboratory or clinical research have remained unsuccessful. Conversely, excessive plasma concentrations of MB can result in reciprocal anticoagulation and unfavorable severe and toxic effects [2].

Administration and Dose

For intravenous administration, MB is dissolved in sterile water to reach a concentration of 1% (10 mg.ml^{-1}). For oral use, it is handled in gelatin capsules to prevent oral mucosa staining and ensure complete absorption through the gastrointestinal tract. Oral doses of up to 300 mg per day or 50 mg TID are reported to be safe in the hereditary methemoglobinemia treatment and the prevention of encephalopathy associated with the chemotherapeutic agent isophosphamide. Moreover, MB is used as a dye in surgical procedures to detect fistulas or leaks from anastomosis procedures and infertility investigations [1].

In adults exhibiting hypotensive vasodilation, the widely accepted dose is 1–2 mg.Kg^{-1}. This is done in boluses lasting 10–20 minutes or 1 hour. In vasoplegic syndrome, continuous infusions are adopted after the preliminary bolus, extending at intervals ranging from 48 to 72 hours. In septicemic patients, therapy with a bolus of 2 mg.Kg^{-1} and continuous infusion lasting 6 hours at a dose of 0.25–1 mg.Kg^{-1} started 2 hours after the initial bolus was reported. In cardiac surgery for the treatment of septic endocarditis, MB was used at a dose of 2 mg.Kg^{-1} in the prime pump before the onset of CPB, followed by intravenous infusion at a dose of 0.5 mg.Kg^{-1} up to 30 minutes after CPB discontinuation, making a total of 3 hours of MB infusion. In anaphylactic shock developed after radiocontrast injection, a single bolus of 1.5–2 mg.Kg^{-1} was effective in re-establishing blood pressure by restoring the vasoconstrictive action of mimetic sympathetic amines [1].

In in vitro endotoxemia models, MB has been shown to suppress PGI-2 production in the presence or absence of proinflammatory cytokines in the human pulmonary smooth muscle cell and canine renal artery. However, with the additional effect on guanylate cyclase, there is the possibility of MB synergistically preventing relaxation induced with NO and PGI-2 in the presence of infection and excessively high local NO concentration [1].

The recognition of the NO role in the hypotension observed in septicemia situations comes from studies that examined the effect of MB on cardiovascular parameters and tissue perfusion in animals. In studies of acute lung injury of ruminants, MB attenuated edema and pulmonary hypertension mediated by endotoxin administration by 50% compared to control. However, the beneficial effects of MB occurred in an early phase of the experiments, being exhausted after 2 hours, with a parallel increase in pulmonary hypertension. Using MB in healthy sheep was associated with an increase in the partial pressure of alveolar-arterial oxygen without the occurrence of hemodynamic changes. The transient improvement in parameters indicative of adequate gas exchange was observed in rabbits submitted to endotoxemia. Such observations indicate the beneficial effect in inhibiting the NO pathway in the presence of the proinflammatory response. However, such inhibition may, at best, result in unaltered hemodynamics and gas exchange, or, at worst, adverse effect of MB when used in conditions unrelated to increased NO production mediated by endotoxin and hypotension. Caution in handling the NO inhibition, maneuver should be mandatory during septicemia, as some studies confirm the occurrence of glomerular thrombosis and liver damage caused by myocardial ischemia. Doubts about MB use have also been elucidated in dogs submitted to endotoxemia, showing manifestations of improvement in pulmonary and systemic hemodynamics, but in a transient manner [2].

NO inhibition as an adjuvant therapy in vasodilatory shock in humans seems naturally attractive once its participation in septic vasodilation is verified. The use of MB in humans with septic shock was associated with an increase in mean arterial pressure (MAP) and systemic vascular resistance (SVR), as well as with the work of the left ventricle, with no change in pulmonary pressure or oxygen exchange. In other studies, the findings of hemodynamic improvement were similar. Also, the heart rate increased; however, the parameters of gas exchange and pulmonary vascular resistance showed worsening of lung function [2].

An increase in ventricular work parallel to the regional decoupling of blood distribution and the potential worsening of pulmonary function implied the cautious use of NO inhibitors in the treatment of vasodilatory shock during septicemia. However, such caution has been questioned in models using continuous MB infusion. The exact role of NO inhibitors remains disputed. In this context, it is essential to note that no study using MB in human patients has been able to reveal an improvement or worsening of survival rates.

Toxicity

Studies have demonstrated that the toxic oral dose in rats is 1180–1250 mg.Kg^{-1} and 40 mg.Kg^{-1} in sheep. In dogs, at a dose of 10–20 mg.Kg^{-1}, hypotension, a drop in systemic vascular resistance (SVR), and decreased renal perfusion are observed.

Data related to teratogenic, carcinogenic, or allergic reactions to MB have not yet been described.

Severe cytotoxicity has been described after the inadvertent use of MB for capsular staining in cataract surgery, causing iris depigmentation and corneal edema evolving to bullous keratopathy and significant vision loss [3].

Ramsay et al. (2007) pointed to the drug interaction between MB and serotonin reuptake inhibitors. MB, characterized as a potent monoamine oxidase (MAO) inhibitor, is administered to patients who are under the treatment of serotonergic drugs responsible for the sudden appearance of toxicity to serotonin [4]. In the United Kingdom, MB must be handled according to the rules of the Control of Substances Harmful to Health. The slightest contact with the eyes and skin can cause irritation and inflammation. Therefore, in case of contact, the area must be washed immediately with water or isotonic saline solution. In humans, toxic manifestations are dose-related and include symptoms such as hemolysis, methemoglobinemia, nausea, vomit, chest pain, dyspnea, and hypertension when doses exceeding 2–7 mg.Kg^{-1} are used. Even higher doses, 20–80 mg.Kg^{-1}, promote refractory hypotension and dermal discoloration.

The use of MB is contraindicated during pregnancy, since, as there is a more significant iNOS expression in the placenta and fetus, it can lead to global or regional hypoxia due to NO inhibition. Its use for the treatment of refractory hypotension in neonates should be done with caution in order not to promote hemolysis and hyperbilirubinemia. Due to the narrow therapeutic index of MB in patients with methemoglobinemia, its use is contraindicated in patients suffering from glucose-6-phosphate dehydrogenase deficiency due to a lower ability to reduce MB to its inactive metabolite, blue leukomethylene. The skin color given by the MB interferes with the pulse oximetry readings, making it impossible to differentiate between dermal discoloration, cyanosis, or desaturation [5].

Given all the concepts discussed, the use of MB seems, at the moment, the most reasonable therapeutic proposal since it does not interfere with NO synthesis, and because it is a medication widely used in other clinical conditions. The action of MB implies inhibition of guanylate cyclase, preventing the elevation of cGMP, and, consequently, avoiding NO-mediated endothelium relaxation (Fig. 8.1).

MB use in patients with septic shock, in the infusion of 1–2 mg.Kg^{-1}, is already established, providing an increase in blood pressure by inhibiting the action of NO in vascular smooth muscle. The NO release has been implicated in the cardiovascular changes of septicemic shock. Since guanylate cyclase is the endothelium-dependent relaxation enzyme, MB being a potent inhibitor of this enzyme is an essential option for the treatment of vasoplegia in sepsis. A study in humans showed that MB increased MAP and stroke volume in septicemic and shocked patients. The other parameters, obtained through the hemodynamic study at the bedside, did not show significant changes, and in some of the studied patients, the effect was not sustained. For this reason, a new dose was administered in an intravenous bolus of 2 mg.Kg^{-1}of the MB, observing the same initial effects. No adverse side effects were observed. This type of observation, regarding the failure to sustain the initial

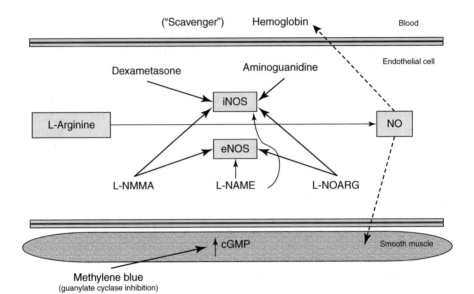

Fig. 8.1 Nitric oxide blockers, highlighting that hemoglobin and methylene blue are independent blockers of synthesis from L-arginine. NO nitric oxide, cGMP guanosine 3′5′-cyclic monophosphate, eNOS endothelial nitric oxide synthase, iNOS inducible nitric oxide synthase, L-NMMA N^G-monomethyl-L-arginine, L-NAME N^G-nitro-L-arginine methyl ester, L-NOARG N^G-nitro-L-arginine

impact, led to the adoption of continuous infusion of MB after the initial intravenous bolus [3].

The clinical use of MB in the treatment of anaphylactic shock, in a literature search, as broad as possible, is found only in the works of Evora et al. [6–8]. The excellent results obtained in 13 clinical cases suggest the fundamental NO role in the pathophysiology of anaphylactic shock, raising MB to a condition of choice, or even priority, in its therapy. The accumulation of clinical experience may confirm these impressions. The MB dosages used (3.0 mg.Kg^{-1}) were adopted based on the knowledge acquired in the treatment of vasoplegia in sepsis and the treatment of methemoglobinemia. This dose is safe since the lethal dose of MB, determined experimentally in goats, is 40 mg.Kg^{-1}.

The catastrophic, and not infrequent, reactions to protamine infusion to neutralize heparin deserve mention. For these cases, experimental and clinical studies attest to the usefulness of MB in the doses already mentioned [6–8].

Finally, this text could not fail to comment on the big "question that does not want to remain silent" on the use of MB: Why does the vasoplegic picture sometimes reverse itself promptly and, sometimes, it seems to do no good?

A brilliant doctoral thesis was defended at the Federal University of Florianópolis, a thesis already published, which brings some extremely important data to try to answer that question [9]. Using a model of sepsis in mice, the authors demonstrated in 24 hours, subdivided into three periods of 8 hours, that there is a dynamic of the guanylate cyclase action in such a way as to create a "window of opportunity" for the MB efficiency in helping to restore systemic vascular resistance. In the first 8 hours, not only the vasocontraction to amines become inefficient, but also the action of NO donor drugs is blunted. This phase coincides with increased iNOS expression. Between 8 and 16 hours, the expression of guanylate cyclase is canceled, probably due to the excess NO production; thus, in this phase, MB would not act. Later, between 16 and 24 hours, there would be a "de novo" guanylate cyclase synthesis, and MB would be useful again [9]. Considering these findings, we started to keep using the MB infusion even without apparent effectiveness, waiting for the "window of opportunity," that is, for the "de novo" guanylate cyclase synthesis (Fig. 8.2). In our experience with patients undergoing cardiopulmonary bypass, we have had the opportunity to test this laboratory evidence. Patients have an excellent response at the end of the cardiopulmonary bypass, but the maintenance of a continuous infusion of MB was associated with the progressive decrease in high doses of noradrenaline and adrenaline [3].

Concluding Remarks

- After exposure to bacterial endotoxin or certain cytokines, the inducible nitric oxide synthase (iNOS) expression occurs in a wide variety of tissues. This enzyme produces large amounts of NO over long periods, closely related to the pathophysiological changes in sepsis.
- The participation of NO overproduction by the iNOS expression is very clear, leading to a state of vasoplegia irresponsible to high doses of catecholamines.
- More knowledge about the NO role in septic shock and the participation of different synthases of nitric oxide, which can be selectively inhibited, is necessary.

Fig. 8.2 "Window of opportunity" for the use of methylene blue relying on the recreation of soluble guanylate cyclase (sGC)

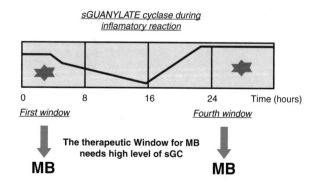

It should be noted that studies in humans had to be interrupted by the observation of an important increase in mortality due to the use of NO synthesis inhibitors.
- Once guanylate cyclase is the endothelium-dependent relaxation enzyme, MB is a potent inhibitor of this enzyme and an important option for the treatment of vasoplegia in sepsis.
- Vasopressin levels in septic shock are abnormally low. This fact supports the hypothesis that in sepsis there may be a decrease in vasopressin stocks and/or a dysfunction of baroreflexes, causing insufficient vasopressin secretion.

References

1. Evora PR, Viaro F. The guanylyl cyclase inhibition by MB as vasoplegic circulatory shock therapeutical target. Curr Drug Targets. 2006;7(9):1195–204.
2. Evora PR, Rodrigues AJ. Methylene blue revised. J Thorac Cardiovasc Surg. 2006;131(1):250–1; author reply 1.
3. Evora PR, Alves Junior L, Ferreira CA, Menardi AC, Bassetto S, Rodrigues AJ, et al. Twenty years of vasoplegic syndrome treatment in heart surgery. Methylene blue revised. Rev Bras Cir Cardiovasc. 2015;30(1):84–92.
4. Ramsay RR, Dunford C, Gillman PK. Methylene blue and serotonin toxicity: inhibition of monoamine oxidase A (MAO A) confirms a theoretical prediction. Br J Pharmacol. 2007;152(6):946–51.
5. Menardi AC, Viaro F, Vicente WV, Rodrigues AJ, Evora PR. Hemodynamic and vascular endothelium function studies in healthy pigs after intravenous bolus infusion of methylene blue. Arq Bras Cardiol. 2006;87(4):525–32.
6. Albuquerque AA, Margarido EA, Menardi AC, Scorzoni AF, Celotto AC, Rodrigues AJ, et al. Methylene blue to treat protamine-induced anaphylaxis reactions. An experimental study in pigs. Braz J Cardiovasc Surg. 2016;31(3):226–31.
7. Oliveira Neto AM, Duarte NM, Vicente WV, Viaro F, Evora PR. Methylene blue: an effective treatment for contrast medium-induced anaphylaxis. Med Sci Monit. 2003;9(11):CS102–6.
8. Evora PR, Roselino CH, Schiaveto PM. Methylene blue in anaphylactic shock. Ann Emerg Med. 1997;30(2):240.
9. Fernandes D, da Silva-Santos JE, Duma D, Villela CG, Barja-Fidalgo C, Assreuy J. Nitric oxide-dependent reduction in soluble guanylate cyclase functionality accounts for early lipopolysaccharide-induced changes in vascular reactivity. Mol Pharmacol. 2006;69(3):983–90.

Chapter 9
The Inhibition of Guanylate Cyclase by Methylene Blue as a Therapeutic Proposal of Vasoplegia Associated with Cardiocirculatory Shock

Guanylate Cyclase

Soluble guanylate cyclase (sGC) is expressed in the cytoplasm of most mammalian cells. It is responsible for mediating a variety of crucial physiological functions such as inhibition of platelet aggregation, smooth muscle relaxation, vasodilation, nerve signal transduction, and immunomodulation. It is the primary enzyme responsible for catalyzing the conversion of guanosine-5′ triphosphate (GTP) to guanosine 3′5′-cyclic monophosphate (cGMP), and it has been described for nearly 40 years after its identification in mammalian cells. Nitric oxide (NO) was described in the late 1970s as responsible for its activation and, therefore, for the formation of cGMP. Ten years later, when the endothelium-derived relaxing factor (EDRF) was discovered and identified as NO, mammalian cells were shown capable of synthesizing this inorganic compound, identifying it then as an endogenous sGC activator. The result was the characterization of the NO-sGC-cGMP transduction system [1–3].

Guanylate cyclase (GC) is designated as soluble or cytosolic to distinguish it from the form bound to the plasma membrane (defined as particulate). The present-day recommendation would be to classify it as sensitive or insensitive to NO. Both are essential for the catalytic exercise of the enzyme. Each subunit displays an N-terminal regulatory domain (where the heme cluster is located), a central dimerization region, and a C-terminal catalytic domain. The sGC shape is composed of two one-of-a-kind subunits known as α, and, in turn, each has two distinct subunits (α1; α2 and β1; β2) [1–3].

Particulate guanylate cyclase differs from soluble in that it is a homomer and has, in addition to the carboxy-terminal catalytic site and dimerization region, a protein kinase homology domain, a transmembrane segment, and an extracellular component for binding enterotoxins and peptides (e.g., atrial natriuretic).

P. R. Barbosa Evora et al., *Vasoplegic Endothelial Dysfunction*, https://doi.org/10.1007/978-3-030-74096-2_9

The N-terminal aspect comprises the prosthetic heme group, whose presence is compulsory for the sGC activation by NO. The heme group is a pentamer ring containing five contributors composed of nitrogen (N), of which four are N atoms coordinated with a central iron (Fe^{+2} reduced form). The fifth, on the other hand, is an axial imidazole ligand coordinated by the subunit β1 using two cysteines adjacent to the His 105 (Cys 78 and Cys 214) using the amino acid histidine at position 105 (His105). The presence of the two subunits is necessary for an adequate orientation of the heme group. However, their coordination is carried out using the N-terminal portion of the β1 subunit using two cysteines adjacent to His 105 (Cys 78 and Cys 214) [1–3].

The heme group gives the sensitivity of the enzyme to NO. NO reacts with this group, forming a penta-coordinated nitrosyl-heme complex that alters the ring configuration. The result is the induction of the activated state of sGC, developing its catalytic activity (GTP in cGMP) up to 200 times. Thus, mutations of the amino acids referred to above lead to the formation of an enzyme that is insensitive to NO.

The catalytic site discovered in the C-terminal component is responsible for the GTP binding. The two subunits, α and β, have their location, but both must be expressed for a catalytic activity to occur. The divalent cations Mn^{+2} and Mg^{+2} are cofactors, and their presence or absence can modulate their activity by enhancing activation or increasing substrate affinity for sGC. The dimerization region is responsible for the union of the two subunits between amino acids 204 and 408.

sGC Activation of the NO Pathway

NO is a free radical that is easy to diffuse and capable of activating sGC by directly linking with the heme group, forming a heme-nitrosyl-ferrous (Fe^{+2}) complex. The half-life of this complex lasts from 4 minutes to 3 hours at a temperature of 20 °C. The oxidation of the heme group to the ferric state (Fe^{+3}) results in the loss of enzymatic activity. Consequently, reducing agents such as thiols or ascorbates increase their activity by maintaining the reduced state, facilitating binding with NO. Conversely, oxidizing agents, such as methylene blue (MB), can inhibit it. The easiest model that describes the NO binding to sGC depends on two phases: (i) NO binding to the heme group, resulting in the formation of a hexa-coordinated complex and (ii) cleavage of the bond between iron and histidine to structure the penta-coordinated nitrosyl-heme. This model emerged after the observation that sGC without a heme group were susceptible to activation by protoporphyrin IX, a compound synthesized from glycine and precursor to heme that structurally resembles penta-coordinated nitrosyl-heme [1–3].

Zao et al. (1999) demonstrated that the transformation dynamics of the hexa-complex to penta-coordinated complex depends on the NO concentration, postulating the existence of a second binding site for NO with a regulatory function on the activity of this enzyme [1]. However, the work of Bellamy et al. (2002) refutes these results by observing that the presence of an additional mechanism is unnecessary since the activation of a single site can predict this activity [2]. Additionally, Cary et al. (2005) elucidated the participation of the ATP and GTP nucleotides in the modulation of the transition from hexa- to penta-coordinated complex, suggesting an even more elaborate model for activating sGC [4].

cGMP and Intracellular Signaling

Guanosine 3′5′-cyclic monophosphate (cGMP) is responsible for regulating several biological functions after sGC activation. Such functions include retinal responses to light stimuli, smell, steroid formation, renal and intestinal ion transport, regulation of intracellular concentration of free calcium (essential for platelet aggregation), and regulation of cardiac, vascular, and nonvascular smooth muscle contractility (springboard for the development of sildenafil – Viagra®). Its dysfunction is related to endotoxemic shock, secretory diarrhea, and hypertension, among others [1–3].

There are three varieties of cGMP receptor intracellular proteins: (1) phosphodiesterases (PDEs), (2) cGMP-sensitive ion channels (CNG), and (3) cGMP-dependent protein kinases (PKG).

The mechanisms by which PKG generates relaxation are not yet fully elucidated but may include (1) reduction in the focus of cytosolic calcium (due to prolonged exports and reduced mobilization mediated by inositol triphosphate IP3) and (2) dephosphorylation of the myosin light chain by activating phosphatases or by maintaining myosin light-chain kinase (MLCK) in the phosphorylated form that is not activated via calmodulin (CaM).

The cellular regulates this Ca^{+2}, which prompts the calcium/calmodulin-dependent myosin light-chain kinase (MLCK), phosphorylating the myosin light chain (MLC) with consequent contraction. The stimulation of sGC by NO causes relaxation, increasing the cGMP production and activating cGMP-dependent protein kinase (PKG) [1–3].

Concluding Remarks

- Soluble guanylate cyclase (GCs) is expressed in the cytoplasm of most mammalian cells and is responsible for mediating a variety of important physiological functions such as inhibition of platelet aggregation, smooth muscle relaxation, vasodilation, transduction of nerve signals, and immunomodulation.
- The sensitivity of the enzyme to nitric oxide (NO) is given by the heme group. NO reacts with this group to form a penta-coordinated nitrosyl-heme complex that alters the ring configuration. The result is the induction of the activated state of GCs, increasing its catalytic activity (GTP in cGMP) by up to 200 times.

- There are three types of cGMP receptor intracellular proteins: (1) phosphodiesterases (PDEs), (2) cGMP-sensitive ion channels (CNG), and (3) cGMP-dependent protein kinases (PKG).

References

1. Zhao Y, Brandish PE, Ballou DP, Marletta MA. A molecular basis for nitric oxide sensing by soluble guanylate cyclase. Proc Natl Acad Sci U S A. 1999;96(26):14753–8.
2. Bellamy TC, Wood J, Garthwaite J. On the activation of soluble guanylyl cyclase by nitric oxide. Proc Natl Acad Sci U S A. 2002;99(1):507–10.
3. Evora PR, Viaro F. The guanylyl cyclase inhibition by MB as vasoplegic circulatory shock therapeutical target. Curr Drug Targets. 2006;7(9):1195–204.
4. Cary SP, Winger JA, Marletta MA. Tonic and acute nitric oxide signaling through soluble guanylate cyclase is mediated by nonheme nitric oxide, ATP, and GTP. Proc Natl Acad Sci U S A. 2005;102(37):13064–9.

Chapter 10
Methylene Blue in the Treatment of Anaphylaxis

The anaphylactic shock (ASh) is one of three types of distributive shock and can now be defined as an acute syndrome and represents the most severe clinical manifestation of allergic diseases. Potentially fatal, it is a type I hypersensitivity reaction against specific antigens, leading to the formation of antibodies (IgE). However, the intensity of ASh is not only influenced by sensitization but also by several other factors such as the practice of physical exercises, psychogenic stress, or even the use of medications such as adrenergic antagonists [1].

Research in the field of immunology has made it possible to understand the process of sensitizing an organism to an allergen. Currently, it is described that anaphylaxis is triggered by the formation of the antigen-antibody immuno-complex on the surface of cells such as mast cells and basophils. The immune response begins when an allergen is absorbed by a macrophage that carries it to a B lymphocyte. It recognizes it and becomes sensitized and quickly turns into a plasma cell. Under the stimulation of the auxiliary lymphocytes, the plasmocytes start to produce large amounts of IgE that are fixed in the mast cells. Thus, a second exposure to the antigen alters the Fc fragment of the high-affinity IgE receptor and induces mast cell degranulation, releasing histamine.

Anaphylactic Shock and Nitric Oxide

Anaphylactic shock (ASh) is classified as a type I hypersensitivity reaction, forming antibodies (IgE). IgE activates the release of histamine from basophils and mast cells. One of the hypotheses that could explain the important vasodilatory effect of histamine in ASh is that histamine binds to H1 receptors in the vascular endothelium, activating the nitric oxide (NO) production, one of the relaxing factors derived from the endothelium, which diffuses to vascular smooth muscle and activates the guanosine 3′5′-cyclic monophosphate (cGMP) production, resulting in

P. R. Barbosa Evora et al., *Vasoplegic Endothelial Dysfunction*, https://doi.org/10.1007/978-3-030-74096-2_10

vasodilation. Histamine can also bind to H2 receptors present in vascular smooth muscle, activating the adenosine 3'5'-cyclic monophosphate (cAMP) production pathway that also results in vasodilation. Thus, the vasodilation resulting from the activation of the cGMP and cAMP pathways synergistically contributes to the development and maintenance of the characteristic ASh hypotension [1].

There are many substances capable of mediating ASh: prostaglandins, leukotrienes, and platelet aggregation factor (PAF). However, histamine appears to be the main secretory product of basophils and mast cells.

Since the mid-1970s of the last century, the presence of H1 and H2 receptors in the pulmonary and systemic circulation has been described, illustrating the importance of histamine in ASh mediation, since when released and transported by the bloodstream, it can produce an effect on the entire cardiovascular system, in addition to other tissues where histaminergic receptors can also be found.

In this sense, experiments carried out on rats, dogs, and humans demonstrated that histamine-mediated vasodilation is dependent on the endothelium, suggesting that histamine induces the release of endothelium-derived relaxing factors (EDRFs). H1 receptors can be found on endothelial cells. These receptors are coupled to the Gq protein that activates the phospholipase C (PLC), inositol 1,4,5-triphosphate (IP3), and diacylglycerol (DAG) pathway, involved in increasing the cytoplasmic Ca^{+2} concentration, which in endothelial cells results in the NO production by activating isoforms constituting the NO synthase enzyme, such as nNOS (neuronal) and eNOS (endothelial) [1].

Amir and English (1991) verified the NO release in ASh induced with compound 48/80. Later, other authors suggested that NO would be the main EDRF released during anaphylaxis [2]. Thus, different studies about ASh pointed to histamine-mediated NO production as possibly the most critical mechanism activated in the cardiovascular manifestations of anaphylaxis, according to Winbery and Lieberman (2002) [3].

Inflammatory cytokines have also been linked to NO production. These cytokines induce the expression and activity of the induced nitric oxide synthase enzyme (iNOS), which can produce large NO amounts in several cell types where this NO synthase isoform is found. Thus, iNOS could be related to ASh or shock in other inflammatory diseases. However, it has been shown that histamine, via H1 receptors, induces increased expression of the eNOS enzyme. Yet, the fact that the eNOS enzyme is expressed does not necessarily mean it is active. In this sense, Gousset-Dupond et al. (2007) found that eNOS is more expressed and more productive when histamine activation occurs [4]. Corroborating these results, Cauwels et al. (2006), using knockout mice for eNOS and iNOS, showed that not iNOS but eNOS would be the isoform activated in ASh in mice [5].

Once the relationship between NO production and ASh seems established, it is necessary to analyze how NO could modulate the severity of ASh hypotension. In this sense, many studies, sometimes controversial in their findings, have been published, reflecting the complexity and difficulty in conducting these studies, especially *in vitro* tests with endothelial cells.

It is well described in the literature that NO activates the enzyme guanylate cyclase that produces cGMP, whose accumulation in vascular smooth muscle cells results in vasodilation. The inhibition of the enzyme guanylate cyclase with methylene blue (MB), which results in less cGMP production and less vasodilation, has been experimentally and clinically demonstrated.

Histamine-induced vasodilation can also be mediated by the activation of H2 receptors found in the plasma membrane of endothelial cells and smooth muscle cells. The H2 receptors are coupled to the G proteins and the cAMP pathway, which activates PKA. In the endothelium, PKA phosphorylates the NO synthase enzyme, resulting in the NO production, or phosphorylate channels for Ca^{+2}, resulting in an increase in cytoplasmic Ca^{+2}, which binds to calmodulin and activates NO production. In the case of vascular smooth muscle, the activation of H2 receptors results in the cAMP production, which activates mechanisms to reduce the cytoplasmic concentration of Ca^{+2}, with the consequent decoupling of contractile proteins, causing the relaxation of vascular smooth muscle, which can contribute to the characteristic hypotension of ASh [1].

The platelet-activating factor (PAF) is implicated in cardiovascular dysfunctions that occur in several shock syndromes, including anaphylaxis. Excessive production of the vasodilator NO causes hypotension and shock, and it is generally accepted that iNOS is responsible for this. However, the NO contribution to PAF-induced anaphylactic shock or shock is still ambiguous. A study involving PAF and anaphylactic shock in conscious rats showed, surprisingly, that the vasodilation depends entirely on NO, not produced by the iNOS action, but by the eNOS action, which is quickly activated through the PI3K pathway. Soluble guanylate cyclase (sGC) is generally considered to be the primary vasodilator mediator of NO. However, although MB partially prevented PAF-mediated shock, neither 1H- (1, 2, 4) oxadiazole (4,3-a) quinoxaline-1-one (ODQ) nor the deficiency of α1sGC was effective. Also, in two different systemic anaphylaxis models, the inhibition of NOS, PI3K, Akt, and eNOS deficiency gave complete protection. In contrast to the unfounded paradigm that the excessive release of NO derived from iNOS, cardiovascular collapse caused by the eNOS action would be the primary vasodilator in anaphylactic shock. In favor of this hypothesis, unlike in sepsis, where the iNOS expression is later, the cardiocirculatory shock in anaphylaxis is hyperacute [1].

Homeostatic Relationship Between Vasoactive Drugs and Nitric Oxide

Anaphylactic hypotension is treated with fluid therapy, epinephrine, and other vasopressors, if necessary. However, some patients with anaphylaxis do not respond to H1 and H2 histamines, along with fluid therapy, amines, and corticosteroids. Even with optimal medical treatment, anaphylactic hypotension can persist for many hours. Such lack of improvement suggests that current treatments do not correct all pathophysiological events associated with the reaction and other mediators that may play an essential role in this clinical syndrome [1–5].

The physiological response to the effective decrease in circulating blood volume in anaphylaxis involves the release of endogenous catecholamines. Adrenaline is indicated for the initial anaphylaxis treatment. Vasopressin and glucagon have been proposed as adjuvant anaphylaxis treatment in patients who have not responded to adrenaline. Glucagon inhibits the iNOS and NO production. Catecholamines activate adenyl cyclase, which results in increased cAMP. Vasopressin and glucagon also cause an increase in cAMP. On the other hand, cAMP inhibits NO production, which in turn decreases the release of catecholamines and the biological activity of norepinephrine. The NOS inhibition also increases the release of catecholamines, suggesting a homeostatic feedback mechanism between agonists that maintains vascular tone. These agonists inhibit NO production, which inhibits both the release and the activity of catecholamines. The physiological result depends on which effect is predominant. Intervention to inhibit the NO effect would result in the effect of the predominant catecholamine.

Treatment of Anaphylaxis by Inhibition of Nitric Oxide Synthesis

NO seems to play an important pathophysiological role in modulating systemic changes associated with anaphylaxis. NOS inhibitors attenuate hypotension and blood concentration and decrease venous return in such conditions, although they do not improve cardiac depression. On the other hand, NO functionally antagonizes the effects of vasoconstrictors released during in vitro anaphylaxis, and there is no experimental evidence that its production can reduce some pathophysiological changes associated with anaphylaxis, except for vasodilation.

The use of NOS inhibitors in experimental anaphylactic shock therapy is questionable. NOS inhibitors can increase blood pressure, but at the same time, there is a marked reduction in cardiac output. Also, the NO produced by the bronchial epithelium can play an essential role in the fight against anaphylactic bronchospasm. Thus, NOS inhibitors can exacerbate bronchoconstriction in anaphylaxis and worsen the clinical condition [2].

Putting these data together, it appears that NOS inhibitors may have a limited role in anaphylactic shock therapy, compared to endotoxic, septic, or hemorrhagic shock, due to differences in pathophysiological mechanisms, the nature of NOS isoforms involved, and differences in clinical presentation.

Treatment of Anaphylaxis by the Inhibition of Guanylate Cyclase

Animal Studies

The successful use of MB in various forms of vasoplegic circulatory shock suggests that reducing cGMP production by inhibiting guanylate cyclase is clinically viable. A study of anaphylactic shock induced by compound 48/80 in rabbits showed that MB prolongs survival and improves blood pressure. Another study with anaphylactic shock caused by compound 48/80 in pigs also demonstrated that MB increases systemic vascular resistance. However, in none of these studies there was a documented difference in plasma nitrate concentration between the control and experimental animal groups.

Clinical Experience

Fifteen patients with anaphylactic hypotension were successfully treated with MB and reported in the literature. Effective dosages ranged from 1.5 to 2.0 mg.Kg^{-1} bolus and/or infusion. Clinical responses occurred in about 20 minutes. This case series suggests that MB is effective in reversing anaphylactic hypotension. MB has also been successfully used to treat patients affected by anaphylactoid reactions induced by protamine and aprotinin [1].

As anaphylaxis and anaphylactic shock are medical emergencies, and, as there is no evidence to propose MB as the drug of choice, it is very difficult or impossible to design a randomized study that would be under ethical principles. Among the total of our ten patients, three did not present circulatory collapse and only showed the main signs of anaphylaxis. It is essential to differentiate the two situations (anaphylaxis and anaphylactic shock), which were reversed by MB, thus emphasizing their use in cases of anaphylactic reactions without cardiovascular collapse [1].

Methylene Blue

Pharmacological studies in sheep have shown that the 24-hour lethal dose of MB is 42.3 mg.Kg^{-1} (95% confidence interval, 37.3–47.9 mg.Kg^{-1}) in this species. Experimental doses of 2.0 and 3 mg/kg in pigs and rabbits resulted in no change in mean arterial pressure in both species. The terminal half-life of MB in healthy people is 5.25 hours. Reports of toxic effects include hemolytic anemia in newborns at doses of 2–4 mg/kg; nausea, vomiting, abdominal pain, fever, and hemolysis with 7 mg.Kg^{-1}; and hypotension at 20 mg.Kg^{-1}. It has also been reported that MB can cause methemoglobinemia. In humans, MB is used at a dose of 5–7.5 mg.Kg^{-1}

during parathyroid surgery to visualize the glands. This dose is generally well tolerated. However, occasional transient neurotoxicity has been reported at these high doses. In Britain, the National Poisons Information Service recommends an intravenous dose of 4 mg.Kg^{-1} or less. Physicians should also be aware that MB interferes with pulse oximetry and causes occasional oxygen unsaturation.

Conclusions

Further studies are needed to assess the role of MB in anaphylaxis. Based on the clinical experience above, we have created a line of research to study experimentally the treatment of anaphylactic shock, which is currently one of our goals. Considering the lack of knowledge, the experimental protocols we started produced satisfactory responses. These observations do not allow MB to be taken as the drug of choice for the anaphylactic shock treatment. Also, it must be emphasized that adrenaline remains the drug of choice. However, it is possible to speculate about the synergism between these two drugs, since this association acts to stimulate the cAMP system and block the cGMP system, thus compensating for vasoplegia. The accumulated experience strongly suggests that MB is a lifesaving treatment for anaphylactic shock or anaphylaxis and other vasoplegic conditions.

Concluding Remarks

- Anaphylactic shock (ASh) is classified as a type I hypersensitivity reaction, forming antibodies (IgE). IgE activates the release of histamine from basophils and mast cells.
- One of the hypotheses that could explain the important vasodilator effect of histamine in ASh is that histamine binds to H1 receptors in the vascular endothelium, activating the nitric oxide (NO) production, one of the relaxing factors derived from the endothelium, which diffuses to vascular smooth muscle and activates the production of guanosine 3'5'-cyclic monophosphate(cGMP), resulting in vasodilation.
- Histamine can also bind to H2 receptors present in vascular smooth muscle, activating the adenosine 3'5'-cyclic monophosphate (cAMP) production pathway that also results in vasodilation. Thus, the vasodilation resulting from the activation of the cGMP and cAMP pathways synergistically contribute to the development and maintenance of the characteristic ASh hypotension.
- The use of NOS inhibitors in experimental anaphylactic shock therapy is questionable. NOS inhibitors can increase blood pressure, but at the same time, there is a marked reduction in cardiac output. Also, the NO produced by the bronchial epithelium can play an essential role in the fight against anaphylactic

bronchospasm. Thus, NOS inhibitors can exacerbate bronchoconstriction in anaphylaxis and worsen the clinical condition.

- MB has also been successfully used to treat patients affected by anaphylactoid reactions induced by protamine and aprotinin.
- As anaphylaxis and anaphylactic shock are medical emergencies and, as there is no evidence to propose MB as the drug of choice, it is very difficult or impossible to design a randomized study that would be under ethical principles.
- Also, it must be emphasized that adrenaline remains the drug of choice. However, it is possible to speculate about the synergism between these two drugs, since this association acts to stimulate the cAMP system and block the cGMP system, thus compensating for vasoplegia. The accumulated experience strongly suggests that MB is a lifesaving treatment for anaphylactic shock or anaphylaxis and other vasoplegic conditions.

References

1. Evora PR, Simon MR. Role of nitric oxide production in anaphylaxis and its relevance for the treatment of anaphylactic hypotension with methylene blue. Ann Allergy Asthma Immunol. 2007;99(4):306–13.
2. Amir S, English AM. An inhibitor of nitric oxide production, N^G-nitro-L-arginine-methyl ester, improves survival in anaphylactic shock. Eur J Pharmacol. 1991;203(1):125–7.
3. Winbery SL, Lieberman PL. Histamine and antihistamines in anaphylaxis. Clin Allergy Immunol. 2002;17:287–317.
4. Gousset-Dupont A, Robert V, Grynberg A, Lacour B, Tardivel S. The effect of n-3 PUFA on eNOS activity and expression in Ea hy 926 cells. Prostaglandins Leukot Essent Fatty Acids. 2007;76(3):131–9.
5. Cauwels A, Janssen B, Buys E, Sips P, Brouckaert P. Anaphylactic shock depends on PI3K and eNOS-derived NO. J Clin Invest. 2006;116(8):2244–51.

Chapter 11
Methylene Blue in Children and Neonates

Hemodynamic shock is a serious occurrence in the pediatric and neonatal population. Approximately 30% of the patients admitted to the neonatal unit receive inotropic support, and hemodynamic instability is an independent predictor of early neonatal mortality.

Shock treatment in neonatal patients remains a challenge, with difficulties ranging from diagnosis to drug use. The drugs currently available for the treatment of shock are overly aggressive, and patients in shock have worse results showing a higher incidence of serious sequelae, for example, intraventricular cerebral hemorrhage [1–6].

The main cause of distributive shock in children, especially neonatal patients, is septic shock. Mortality in sepsis is still high worldwide, and neonates and children with distributive shock are especially susceptible to the undesirable side effects of high-dose catecholamine infusions. However, they can significantly benefit from methylene blue (MB) infusion before catecholamine infusions. Unfortunately, there is a widely publicized concept that MB cannot be used in children and neonates because it causes pulmonary hypertension.

MB has been recommended in refractory shock treatment. Several studies have evaluated the positive inotropic and vasoconstrictor effects of MB on septic shock, anaphylactic shock, toxin-induced shock, and patients with vasoplegic syndrome after myocardial revascularization surgery.

The administration of MB in septic patients is associated with increases in mean arterial pressure, while reducing the dose of catecholamine in patients. Increased pulmonary vascular resistance has been reported with bolus administration but can be prevented by continuous infusion. No other harmful effects have been reported. The effects on mortality have not been adequately assessed [1–6].

Although the use of MB in pediatric patients is better described, the use in neonatal patients is still controversial. The first report on the use of MB in neonatal patients was in 1951, in a series of cases of eight premature infants, for the treatment of methemoglobinemia. Other uses reported for MB in neonates were for diagnostic

P. R. Barbosa Evora et al., *Vasoplegic Endothelial Dysfunction*, https://doi.org/10.1007/978-3-030-74096-2_11

tests for toxoplasmosis and anatomical gastrointestinal defects. Its use in the treatment of vasoplegia in neonates was described in 1996. The drug was administered to five patients with refractory shock, using dopamine and adrenaline, resulting in increased pressure.

Although studies with MB show favorable results, this drug is little used and mainly in children of pediatric age. MB is an inexpensive, available, safe, and possibly effective adjunct medication in pediatric patients. Therefore, the objective of the present review is to present baseline data for the use of MB in pediatric and neonatal patients.

Evidence of the Role of the L-Arginine/Nitric Oxide Pathway in Neonatal Vascular Reactivity

There are several roles of the L-arginine/nitric oxide/cGMP pathway in pediatric and neonatal patients. There are reports of action in closing the ductus arteriosus at the beginning of the day of other actions, all related to vasoreactivity for adaptation in the extrauterine life after birth.

Two cases reported by Fakler et al. (1995) suggest that the nitric oxide (NO) production from L-arginine may play a role in the normal regulation of systemic blood pressure. Infants with arginine succinate lyase deficiency, who were unable to synthesize L-arginine, were hypertensive before arginine replacement. The infusion of L-arginine resulted in a decrease in blood pressure [7].

Regarding the presence in the neonatal respiratory tract, Sheffield et al. (2006) evaluated nitric oxide synthase (NOS) isoforms in the vascular tree in neonatal lungs at different gestational ages. NOS isoforms were found in the epithelium of the airways (bronchus, alveolus, and more distal air space), and the NOS ontogeny does not show significant changes in abundance or distribution with advancing gestational age or with chronic lung disease [8].

Respiratory distress syndrome (RDS) is quite common in neonates. One of the characteristics of this disease is the increase in carbon dioxide (CO_2), and there is a relationship between carbon dioxide and elevation of guanosine $3'5'$-cyclic monophosphate (cGMP). In 2004, 52 babies (without RDS, $n = 21$; RDS, $n = 31$) were studied. Infants with RDS had higher levels of cGMP compared to those without RDS, and multiple linear regression analysis showed a significant correlation between cGMP and CO_2, suggesting a causal relationship. The authors concluded that an increase in CO_2 caused systemic vasodilation due to the increase in cGMP, with consequent lower blood pressure and greater need for pressure support in premature babies with RDS [6, 9, 10].

Regarding pulmonary arterial pressure, cGMP plays an important role, favoring pulmonary vasodilation. A prospective study, with 18 newborns with high pulmonary pressure diagnosed with Doppler and treated with NO, was investigated. There was a significant increase in plasma cGMP after 60 minutes of NO therapy, and this effect was accompanied by changes in the oxygenation index and a decrease in pulmonary artery pressure.

Poorly controlled brain circulation is also a feature of premature infants. It is suggested that the excessive production of NO predisposes to peri-/intraventricular hemorrhage (PIVH) in the immature newborn. van Bel et al. (2002) studied 83 premature newborns. NO production was assessed by measuring plasma cGMP at 0, 24, 48, 72, and 168 hours of age. Simultaneously, cranial ultrasound investigations were performed, and hemodynamic variables were recorded. The logistic regression model revealed that cGMP was significantly associated with PIVH, regardless of gestational age, mean arterial pressure, or severity of infant respiratory distress syndrome. The authors concluded that impaired cerebral self-regulation induced by vasodilator NO played a role in PIHV [11].

The L-arginine/NOS/cGMP pathway also plays an important role in neonatal septic shock. NO formed by the enzyme NO synthase (NOS) of L-arginine is an important mediator for the elimination of pathogens. Being a potent NO vasodilator is implicated in hypotension and decreased organ perfusion in sepsis. Aydemir et al. (2015) studied 31 neonates with sepsis and 20 controls. L-arginine levels were higher in neonates with septic shock compared to septic neonates without shock ($p = 0.012$) and controls ($p < 0.001$) [12].

Therefore, there is much evidence of the action of the L-arginine/nitric oxide pathway on neonatal vascular reactivity, thus supporting the use of drugs that act on these specific pathways in neonatal and pediatric patients. However, further studies are needed to understand the mechanism and hemodynamic effects of MB.

Adult Methylene Blue Experience

Our institution has substantial experience with MB in the treatment of vasoplegic syndrome related to cardiac surgery. Some observations in adults would apply to children: (1) The use of MB did not cause endothelial dysfunction; (2) the MB effect appears in cases without positive regulation of NO; (3) MB itself is not a vasoconstrictor: by blocking the cGMP pathway, it releases the adenosine 3'5'-cyclic monophosphate(cAMP) pathway, facilitating the vasoconstrictor effect of epinephrine through this "crosstalk" mechanism; (5) the most used dosage is 2 mg.Kg^{-1} in intravenous (IV) bolus, followed by the same continuous hourly infusion, as the plasma concentration declines sharply in the first 40 minutes. These concepts can be applied to neonatal and pediatric patients [13, 14].

Methylene Blue to Treat Vasoplegic Dysfunction in Children

The use of MB in pediatric and neonatal patients has been little studied. In addition, there is no consensus in the literature on the best way to manage MB. The best form of infusion (bolus or continuous), the initial dose, and the progression of the dose are not known; only the maximum dose is recommended (2 mg/Kg/dose). Also, there are no studies on the administration time (hours or days). Therefore, studies are needed to assess these unanswered questions about MB.

Side Effects and Security

When used in therapeutic doses (<2 mg.Kg^{-1}), MB is a safe medication. Leyh et al. observed cardiac arrhythmias; coronary vasoconstriction; decreased cardiac output, renal blood flow, and mesenteric blood flow; increased pulmonary pressure and vascular resistance; and deterioration gas exchange as adverse effects of MB in the treatment of vasoplegia refractory to norepinephrine. However, they concluded that most side effects were dose dependent, not present at 2 mg.Kg^{-1}or less, and reported no side effects with the use of MB (2 mg.Kg^{-1}) in 54 patients [15].

In pediatric studies, the authors did not observe significant side effects in pediatric patients with a dose lower than 2 mg.Kg^{-1}, except for the change in urine color to blue-green in all patients. On the other hand, in some cases there was a significant increase in pulmonary pressure after the MB infusion, being more prominent in cases of atrial and interatrial communication (ASD-VSD). Nevertheless, the increase in pulmonary pressure did not reach clinical significance, and the occurrence was assumed through indirect measures, such as increased right ventricular pressure.

Flyn et al. (2009) reported the reversal of vasodilator shock in a pediatric lung transplant patient without deleterious effects of the note. It is possible, but not proven, that the concomitant use of inhaled NO decreased the chance of adverse pulmonary vasoconstriction in the present patient. It remains to be studied whether the use of inhaled NO offers adequate protection against increases in pulmonary vasoconstriction in patients who would suffer harmful consequences from these increases. With the recognition of the possible risks of MB and the use of preventive measures such as inhaled NO to protect the pulmonary vasculature, MB can be a lifesaver in pediatric patients. The use of MB in pediatric and neonatal patients has been little studied. In addition, there is no consensus in the literature on the best way to manage MB. The best form of infusion (bolus or continuous), the initial dose, and the progression of the dose are not known, only the maximum recommended dose (2 mg/kg/dose) [15].

Conclusion

The action of the L-arginine/nitric oxide pathway in pediatric and neonatal patients is documented, mainly as a mechanism of hemodynamic instability; however, there is a lack of research on the use of MB in this group of patients, and, mainly, in case report studies, there are no side effects of MB in this population that contraindicate its use, and currently this drug is released for use in children. There is evidence that MB can be a useful medication in neonatal and pediatric hemodynamic management, as it has the potential to minimize the use of traditional vasoactive amines, known to cause a deleterious effect in these patients. Therefore, MB, little studied in pediatrics, can prove to be a beneficial medicine in pediatrics and further studies should be performed.

Concluding Remarks

- The main cause of distributive shock in children, especially neonatal patients, is septic shock.
- Mortality in sepsis is still high worldwide, and neonates and children with distributive shock are especially susceptible to the undesirable side effects of high-dose catecholamine infusions.
- However, they can significantly benefit from MB infusion before catecholamine infusions.
- Unfortunately, there is a widely publicized concept that MB cannot be used in children and neonates because it causes pulmonary hypertension.
- There is much evidence of the action of the L-arginine/nitric oxide pathway on neonatal vascular reactivity, thus supporting the use of drugs that act on these specific pathways in neonatal and pediatric patients; however, further studies are needed to understand the mechanism and hemodynamic effects of the MB.
- In pediatric studies, the authors did not observe significant side effects in pediatric patients with a dose lower than 2 mg.Kg^{-1}, except for the change in urine color to blue-green in all patients.
- The use of MB in pediatric and neonatal patients has been little studied. In addition, there is no consensus in the literature on the best way to manage MB. The best form of infusion (bolus or continuous), the initial dose, and the progression of the dose are not known; only the maximum dose is recommended (2 mg/kg/dose).
- There is evidence that MB can be a useful medication in neonatal and pediatric hemodynamic management, as it has the potential to minimize the use of traditional vasoactive amines, known to cause a deleterious effect in these patients. Therefore, MB, little studied in pediatrics, can prove to be a beneficial medicine in pediatrics and further studies should be performed.

References

1. Zakariya BP, Bhat BV, Harish BN, Arun Babu T, Joseph NM. Risk factors and predictors of mortality in culture proven neonatal sepsis. Indian J Pediatr. 2012;79(3):358–61.
2. Femitha P, Bhat BV. Early neonatal outcome in late preterms. Indian J Pediatr. 2012;79(8):1019–24.
3. Al-Aweel I, Pursley DM, Rubin LP, Shah B, Weisberger S, Richardson DK. Variations in prevalence of hypotension, hypertension, and vasopressor use in NICUs. J Perinatol: official journal of the California Perinatal Association. 2001;21(5):272–8.
4. Laughon M, Bose C, Allred E, O'Shea TM, Van Marter LJ, Bednarek F, et al. Factors associated with treatment for hypotension in extremely low gestational age newborns during the first postnatal week. Pediatrics. 2007;119(2):273–80.
5. Noori S, Friedlich PS, Seri I. Pathophysiology of shock in the fetus and neonate. In: Polin RA, Fox WW, Abman SH, editors. Fetal and neonatal physiology. 4th ed. Philadelphia: Elsevier Saunders; 2011. p. 853–63.
6. Bhat BV, Plakkal N. Management of shock in neonates. Indian J Pediatr. 2015;82(10):923–9.
7. Fakler CR, Kaftan HA, Nelin LD. Two cases suggesting a role for the L-arginine nitric oxide pathway in neonatal blood pressure regulation. Acta Paediatr. 1995;84(4):460–2.
8. Sheffield M, Mabry S, Thibeault DW, Truog WE. Pulmonary nitric oxide synthases and nitrotyrosine: findings during lung development and in chronic lung disease of prematurity. Pediatrics. 2006;118(3):1056–64.
9. Cox DJ, Groves AM. Inotropes in preterm infants – evidence for and against. Acta Paediatr. 2012;101(464):17–23.
10. Singh Y, Katheria AC, Vora F. Advances in diagnosis and management of hemodynamic instability in neonatal shock. Front Pediatr. 2018;6:2.
11. van Bel F, Valk L, Uiterwaal CS, Egberts J, Krediet TG. Plasma guanosine 3′,5′-cyclic monophosphate and severity of peri/intraventricular haemorrhage in the preterm newborn. Acta Paediatr. 2002;91(4):434–9.
12. Aydemir O, Ozcan B, Yucel H, Bas AY, Demirel N. Asymmetric dimethylarginine and L-arginine levels in neonatal sepsis and septic shock. J Matern Fetal Neonatal Med. 2015;28(8):977–82.
13. Evora PR, Ribeiro PJ, Vicente WV, Reis CL, Rodrigues AJ, Menardi AC, et al. Methylene blue for vasoplegic syndrome treatment in heart surgery: fifteen years of questions, answers, doubts and certainties. Rev Bras Cir Cardiovasc. 2009;24(3):279–88.
14. Evora PR, Alves Junior L, Ferreira CA, Menardi AC, Bassetto S, Rodrigues AJ, et al. Twenty years of vasoplegic syndrome treatment in heart surgery. Methylene blue revised. Rev Bras Cir Cardiovasc. 2015;30(1):84–92.
15. Flynn BC, Sladen RN. The use of methylene blue for vasodilatory shock in a pediatric lung transplant patient. J Cardiothorac Vasc Anesth. 2009;23(4):529–30.

Chapter 12
Methylene Blue and Burns

The guanylate cyclase inhibition by methylene blue (MB): (1) has been proven, in basic and clinical studies, as an adjuvant treatment option in cases of catecholamine-resistant vasoplegia; (2) its use is safe and generally lifesaving; and (3) the pharmacological inhibition of nitric oxide (NO) interferes not only in the reversal of vasoplegia but also in vascular permeability, often caused by the systemic inflammatory response associated with burns. This review text has three main objectives: (1) to study the guanylate cyclase inhibition by MB in burns; (2) suggest MB as a viable, safe, and useful coadjuvant therapeutic tool for fluid resuscitation; and (3) recommend MB as treatment of hypotensive vasoplegia amine resistant fusion in two burned patients refractory to norepinephrine [1]. The patients had severe burns, 95% and 80% of total body surface area (TBSA), not responding to conventional treatment. Fluid requirements were estimated according to the Parkland formula and then to maintain a urine output of 30–50 mL.h^{-1} [2].

Patient #1 had 95% TBSA and adrenal insufficiency, and was receiving steroids according to the Annane protocol, in addition to vasopressin at 0.2 U/min. His norepinephrine requirements were 55 mcg/kg/min.

Patient #2 had 80% TBSA and was receiving 20 mcg/kg/min of norepinephrine. Circulatory failure was defined as an inability to maintain MAP >70 mmHg. Hemodynamic and physiological parameters were measured before and after the infusion of a single dose of 2 mg.Kg^{-1} of MB. Both patients showed dramatic improvements in their shock after MB. Patient #1 had an initial response in 30 minutes and reached its maximum effect in 1 hour. Noradrenaline requirements decreased to 0.2 mcg kg/min and vasopressin decreased to 0.04 U/min. Patient #2 showed effects within 15 minutes after the infusion, and for 2 hours, norepinephrine was stopped. No adverse effects were observed in these two patients [2].

P. R. Barbosa Evora et al., *Vasoplegic Endothelial Dysfunction*, https://doi.org/10.1007/978-3-030-74096-2_12

Systemic NO Production After Burn Injury

The first investigation to address the issue of NO and thermal injury was reported in Becker et al. (1993). In that study, the urinary level of the stable NO metabolite, NO3, was elevated for 1–8 days in rats subjected to a significant total burned surface area (TBSA) burn injury. It has also been shown that this effect can be prevented by administering the nonspecific nitric oxide synthesis (NOS) inhibitor, N^G-monomethyl-1-arginine (L-NMMA) [3].

In the following year, similar findings were reported by Carter et al. (1994), and an attempt was made to identify the main organs that produce NO by measuring the NOS activity in the tissue. The brain, liver, kidney, spleen, and gastrointestinal tract were seen to have increased NOS activity levels after heat insults. Also, it was observed that the thermally damaged skin is more dependent on calcium. As in previous reports, the results obtained showed a significant increase in plasma NO/NOS levels in burned patients [4].

NO is a central mediator of many physiological and pathophysiological events. After a thermal injury, an increase in NO was observed in the plasma and urinary levels, but the real importance of this fact is unknown. Plasma concentrations of stable NO derivatives (NO^{2-}/NO^{3-}) were determined in 27 burned patients admitted to the Burn Unit at Hospital Santa Maria in Lisbon on days 1, 3, 5, 7, 9, and 15, and their values were compared with healthy controls [5]. A significant increase was found in the determinations of patients burned on admission. Patients with inhalation injury had higher values than the others, with statistical significance on the 5th day. The patients who died showed an increase in NO, with significance on day 5. The determinations in patients with sepsis were higher than in other patients on day 3. No association was found with TBSA. A significant increase in NO was found in burned patients who died between patients with inhalation injury and patients with sepsis. We suggest a possible role for NO determination as a sepsis indicator and the use of NOS inhibitors in these situations.

Nitric Oxide and Vascular Permeability in Burns

Some studies have linked NO production to increased vascular permeability after burn trauma. Sozumi et al. (1997) studied the kinetics and NO role in vascular permeability using a thermal ear injury model. Vascular permeability was suppressed for 3 hours after a thermal injury by the preventive administration of NOS inhibitors. The NO content in the injured region increased significantly compared to the intact area. The authors found that the plasma NO content increased substantially in a biphasic pattern 1 and 6 hours after the injury. NOS inhibitors administered as treatment suppressed vascular permeability 1 and 6 hours after burning, concluding that NOS inhibitors may be useful in the treatment of burns [6].

Inoue et al. (2001) investigated the role of NO and related synthase in thermal injury using experimental burn models to assess the severity of the vascular permeability aspect. Thermal lesions were produced in the murine right ear, pinching with a pair of preheated tweezers. Immediately afterward, Evans' blue dye was administered intravenously, and the mice injured with burns were sacrificed at various times. The burnt ears were collected and hydrolyzed, and the level of extracted dye was measured as an indicator of inflammation. Vascular hyperpermeability was suppressed by the administration of NOS inhibitors. N^G-Nitro-L-Arginine Methyl Ester (L-NAME) not only suppressed vascular hyperpermeability in thermal lesions in a dose-dependent manner but was also effective with prophylactic or therapeutic administration. Although aminoguanidine also suppressed the inflammatory response, it did not affect the initial inflammatory phase. Aminoguanidine, a specific inducible nitric oxide synthase (iNOS) inhibitor, suppressed the late phase, 6 hours after the injury, suggesting that iNOS is involved in the inflammatory responses to thermal lesions. These results also demonstrated that the NOS-type inducible protein stained the burn area immunohistochemically. Therefore, both types of NO mediating enzymes affect inflammatory responses and vascular hyperpermeability, and their regulation may lead to the development of a new therapy for thermal injuries [7].

Resuscitation with Methylene Blue and Volume

Jeroukhimov et al. (2001) conducted an interesting investigation to compare prehospital hypotensive resuscitation with volume resuscitation and find out whether reagents that inhibit the formation of oxygen free radicals, such as MB, can improve resuscitation and survival. After 30 minutes of controlled bleeding, rats were subjected to 60 minutes of uncontrolled bleeding with simultaneous resuscitation. Hartmann's solution alone, or blood or MB bolus, was infused to maintain mean arterial pressure (MAP) at 80 or 40 mmHg. Then the bleeding was stopped, and Hartmann's solution and whole blood were infused to obtain a MAP within normal limits. During uncontrolled hemorrhage, it was not possible to achieve a MAP of 80 mmHg in animals resuscitated only with Hartmann's solution, and all died. All rats that received Hartmann's solution or whole blood associated with an MB bolus achieved a higher MAP. About 40 mmHg of MAP was obtained in all animals, regardless of the resuscitation fluid. Only 15 of the 24 animals were resuscitated to a MAP of 80 mmHg survived, compared with 22 survivors of the 24 rats resuscitated to a MAP of 40 mmHg. MB or whole blood drastically reduced the volumes of spilled blood and fluids and moderated the reduction in compressed cell volume, especially during hypotensive resuscitation. The authors concluded that hypotensive protocols should be used to increase survival. The MB supplied with electrolyte solutions can negate its harmful effects during resuscitation [8].

Precautions for the Use of Methylene Blue

In general, the administration of MB is safe at 2 mg.Kg^{-1} in bolus, but certain risks must be considered. MB has monoamine oxidase inhibitors side effects and, theoretically, can cause serotonin syndrome in patients undergoing selective serotonin reuptake.

Moreover, there have been reports of anaphylaxis resulting from the administration of MB. Perhaps the most important for this patient population is to consider that MB is an inhibitor of vasodilatory effects of NO but also can lead to pulmonary vasoconstriction and impaired gas exchange. However, a prospective study of ten patients administered MB at 1 mg.Kg^{-1} did not show evidence of impaired gas exchange, even in those with lung injury [9]. In fact, animal studies suggest MB has lung protection effects, and when used in conjunction with inhaled NO, it can prevent endotoxin-mediated pulmonary dysfunction. Further study could elucidate whether this therapy could potentially benefit patients with vasoplegia and inhalation injury.

Concluding Remarks

- The guanylate cyclase inhibition by methylene blue: (1) has been proven, in basic and clinical studies, as an adjuvant treatment option in cases of catecholamine-resistant vasoplegia; (2) its use is safe and generally lifesaving; and (3) the pharmacological inhibition of nitric oxide (NO) interferes, not only in the reversal of vasoplegia but also in vascular permeability, often caused by the systemic inflammatory response associated with burns.
- Some studies have linked NO production to increased vascular permeability after burn trauma. Sozumi et al. studied the kinetics and role of NO in vascular permeability using a thermal ear injury model. Vascular permeability was suppressed for 3 hours after a thermal injury by the preventive administration of nitric oxide synthase (NOS) inhibitors.

References

1. Jaskille AD, Jeng JC, Jordan MH. Methylene blue in the treatment of vasoplegia following severe burns. J Burn Care Res. 2008;29(2):408–10.
2. Farina Junior JA, Celotto AC, da Silva MF, Evora PR. Guanylate cyclase inhibition by methylene blue as an option in the treatment of vasoplegia after a severe burn. A medical hypothesis. Med Sci Monit. 2012;18(5):HY13–7.
3. Becker WK, Shippee RL, McManus AT, Mason AD Jr, Pruitt BA Jr. Kinetics of nitrogen oxide production following experimental thermal injury in rats. J Trauma. 1993;34(6):855–62.

4. Carter EA, Derojas-Walker T, Tamir S, Tannenbaum SR, Yu YM, Tompkins RG. Nitric oxide production is intensely and persistently increased in tissue by thermal injury. Biochem J. 1994;304(Pt 1):201–4.

5. do Rosario Caneira da Silva M, Mota Filipe H, Pinto RM, de Salaverria Timoteo C, Godinho de Matos MM, Cordeiro Ferreira A, et al. Nitric oxide and human thermal injury short term outcome. Burns. 1998;24(3):207–12.

6. Sozumi T. The role of nitric oxide in vascular permeability after a thermal injury. Ann Plast Surg. 1997;39(3):272–7.

7. Inoue H, Ando K, Wakisaka N, Matsuzaki K, Aihara M, Kumagai N. Effects of nitric oxide synthase inhibitors on vascular hyperpermeability with thermal injury in mice. Nitric Oxide. 2001;5(4):334–42.

8. Jeroukhimov I, Weinbroum A, Ben-Avraham R, Abu-Abid S, Michowitz M, Kluger Y. Effect of methylene blue on resuscitation after haemorrhagic shock. Eur J Surg Acta chirurgica. 2001;167(10):742–7.

9. Andresen M, Dougnac A, Diaz O, Hernandez G, Castillo L, Bugedo G, et al. Use of methylene blue in patients with refractory septic shock: impact on hemodynamics and gas exchange. J Crit Care. 1998;13(4):164–8.

Chapter 13
Cardiac Arrest and Neuroprotection by Methylene Blue

Some Pathophysiology Data

After the onset of cardiac arrest, global ischemia activates the glia and the complement system with the release of cytokines by neurons. The pro-inflammatory cascade is initiated by the expression of adhesion molecules, polymorphonuclear leukocyte chemotaxis, and the reactive oxygen species production. As a result, there is an increase in vascular permeability, blood clotting activation, platelet activation, and vasoconstrictors release, contributing to the regional flow reduction. Cerebral edema increased blood-brain barrier (BBB) permeability and neurological damage are seen early in ischemia-induced by cardiac arrest. The positive nitric oxide synthase (NOS) regulation is associated with an increase in nitric oxide (NO) production that induces the BBB breakdown. It has been suggested that pretreatment with pharmacological agents can reduce excess NO or oxidative stress, decreasing the interruption of BBB permeability caused by ischemia/reperfusion injury. Methylene blue (MB), a nontoxic dye and scavenger cleaner, recently proved to be a potential aid in the resuscitation of cardiac arrest, attenuating oxidative, inflammatory, myocardial, and neurological lesions [1].

Stocks of Methylene Blue

In the central nervous system (CNS), MB is a protector against various insults, and, based on its effect on mitochondrial cytochrome oxidase, it has been proposed as a cerebral metabolic enhancer [2].

MB has a wide range of targets, covering various neurotransmitter systems, ion channels, and enzymes involved in multiple physiological functions of the nervous system. It appears that many of the biological effects of MB are strongly associated

P. R. Barbosa Evora et al., *Vasoplegic Endothelial Dysfunction*, https://doi.org/10.1007/978-3-030-74096-2_13

with its unique physicochemical properties, including its redox characteristics, ionic charges, and characteristics of the light spectrum. MB has a high solubility in an aqueous medium; preclinical and clinical studies suggest low toxicity. Also, its ability to penetrate cell membranes and cross the blood-brain barrier (BBB) makes MB attractive as a potential therapeutic agent. However, as pointed out by Oz et al. (2001), there are still many open questions about the impact of MB on CNS disorders, and further studies are needed to elucidate the molecular and cellular targets of MB's actions. Perhaps this is the best criticism on the subject, and its reading is mandatory [3].

Among Methylene Blue's Actions, Three of Them Deserve Attention for Neuroprotection

1. *The therapeutic effects of MB are attributed to the presence of the nitric oxide/ guanosine 3'5'-cyclic monophosphate (NO/cGMP) signaling system and its impact on iron-containing enzymes. Thus, MB has its controversial direct inhibitory effects on NO synthases and also blocks cGMP synthesis, inhibiting the enzyme soluble guanylate cyclase.*
2. *MB, an alternative electron carrier, can accept electrons from NADH. Therefore, MB can prevent electron leakage and increase mitochondrial oxidative phosphorylation, reducing the overproduction of free radicals under pathological conditions. When restoring mitochondrial function, MB is a powerful neuroprotection in many neurological disorders (e.g., Alzheimer's and Parkinson's disease). The inhibition of MB xanthine oxidase also protects against the toxic effects of some free oxygen radicals.*
3. *MB inhibits Tau (a phosphoprotein) phosphorylation and plays an essential role in regulating its physiological function. In neurodegenerative disorders such as Alzheimer's disease (AD), corticobasal degeneration, or supranuclear palsy, the Tau protein is an abnormally phosphorylated neurofibrillary tangle which correlates with dementia and pyramidal cell damage.*

Experimental investigations have proven the cardioprotective and neuroprotective effects of MB in a *swine* model of experimental cardiac arrest. The main physiological effects during reperfusion include: (1) systemic stabilization of the circulation without significantly increasing the total peripheral resistance; (2) a moderate increase in cerebral cortical blood flow; (3) reduction of peroxidation and lipid inflammation; and (4) less anoxic damage to the brain and heart tissue [4].

An intriguing investigation studied the effects of cardiac arrest and cardiopulmonary resuscitation (CPR) on BBB permeability and consequent neurological damage. This investigation studied the MB effects on maintaining the BBB integrity and the NO release in the cerebral cortex. In a 12-minute porcine model of cardiac arrest, the authors demonstrated a transient increase in necrotic neurons, caused by ischemia and reperfusion. Also, the immunohistochemical analysis indicated less rupture of the blood-brain barrier in animals that received MB, evidenced by the decrease in extra leakage of albumin, water, and potassium content and less neuronal damage. Likewise, treatment with MB reduced the nitrite/nitrate ratio, inducible nitric oxide synthase (iNOS) expression, and neuronal nitric oxide synthase (nNOS) expression. In summary, MB markedly reduced the BBB and the subsequent neurological injury. In addition to these cerebral morphological effects, exposure to MB is associated with a decrease of NO content as measured by nitrate/nitrite and the partial inhibition of NOS activity [4, 5].

Mild hypothermia induced neuroprotective effects on CPR. However, inducing hypothermia is time-consuming. A study showed that the MB administered during CPR could increase the neuroprotective effect of hypothermia. In cardiac arrest with variable duration of CPR, it was demonstrated that the neuroprotective effect of MB in combination with hypothermia was significantly higher than late hypothermia alone. Also, a porcine model of cardiac arrest, without comparing 12 minutes without CPR and 8 minutes with CPR, was used to evaluate the addition of MB to hypertonic saline, dextran solution. Hemodynamic variables were slightly improved at 15 minutes and MB, co-administered with a hypertonic-hyperoncotic solution, increased survival in 4 hours, reducing neurological damage. MB can also be used in combination with hypertonic sodium chloride solution, but it precipitates. However, an alternative mixture of MB in hypertonic sodium lactate was developed and investigated, using the same piglet model, during and after CPR. This association could be used against reperfusion injury during experimental cardiac arrest, with effects similar to MB in dextran hypertonic saline [6].

There are no publications considering MB, vasoplegia, and neuroprotection, but the above concepts would be relevant considering the protection of the brain in cardiac surgery.

Concluding Remarks

- The positive nitric oxide synthase (NOS) regulation is associated with an increase in nitric oxide (NO) production that induces the blood-brain barrier (BBB) breakdown.
- It has been suggested that pretreatment with pharmacological agents can reduce excess NO or oxidative stress, decreasing the interruption of BBB permeability caused by ischemia/reperfusion injury.
- Methylene blue (MB), a nontoxic dye and also a scavenger cleaner, recently proved to be a potential aid in the resuscitation of cardiac arrest, attenuating oxidative, inflammatory, myocardial, and neurological lesions.
- MB has a wide range of targets, covering various neurotransmitter systems, ion channels, and enzymes involved in various physiological functions of the nervous system.
- MB has its controversial direct inhibitory effects on NO synthases and blocks guanosine 3'5'-cyclic monophosphate (cGMP) synthesis, inhibiting the enzyme

soluble guanylate cyclase. MB inhibits Tau (which is a phosphoprotein) phosphorylation and plays an important role in regulating its physiological function.
- MB could also be used in combination with hypertonic sodium chloride, but it precipitates.

References

1. Batista-Filho MM, Kandratavicius L, Nunes EA, Tumas V, Colli BO, Hallak JE, et al. Role of methylene blue in trauma neuroprotection and neuropsychiatric diseases. CNS Neurol Disord Drug Targets. 2016;15(8):976–86.
2. Baldo CF, Silva LM, Arcencio L, Albuquerque AAS, Celotto AC, Basile-Filho A, et al. Why methylene blue have to be always present in the stocking of emergency antidotes. Curr Drug Targets. 2018;19(13):1550–9.
3. Oz M, Lorke DE, Hasan M, Petroianu GA. Cellular and molecular actions of methylene blue in the nervous system. Med Res Rev. 2011;31(1):93–117.
4. Wiklund L, Basu S, Miclescu A, Wiklund P, Ronquist G, Sharma HS. Neuro- and cardioprotective effects of blockade of nitric oxide action by administration of methylene blue. Ann N Y Acad Sci. 2007;1122:231–44.
5. Miclescu A, Sharma HS, Martijn C, Wiklund L. Methylene blue protects the cortical blood-brain barrier against ischemia/reperfusion-induced disruptions. Crit Care Med. 2010;38(11):2199–206.
6. Miclescu A, Basu S, Wiklund L. Cardio-cerebral and metabolic effects of methylene blue in hypertonic sodium lactate during experimental cardiopulmonary resuscitation. Resuscitation. 2007;75(1):88–97.

Chapter 14
Methylene Blue and Endocarditis

Infective endocarditis (IE) is a life-threatening condition that occasionally requires emergency valve replacement. Patients with an ongoing systemic inflammatory response because of infective endocarditis and those who need cardiopulmonary bypass (CPB) for emergency valve replacement may demonstrate resistant hypotension related to vasoplegia. It presents a spectrum of clinical presentation and is associated with a systemic inflammatory response and the release of endothelial nitric oxide (NO). Hemodynamically it is characterized by arterial vasodilation, high cardiac output despite myocardial depression, and decreased sensitivity of the heart and peripheral vessels to sympathomimetic agents.

Grayling et al. (2003) described the first case of methylene blue (MB) used in the CPB prime and in the context of refractory hypotension in a patient undergoing valve replacement surgery for infective endocarditis, suggesting that MB should be added to the CPB prime (2 mg.Kg^{-1}) and continued as an infusion (0.25–2 mg/(kg h)) to improve this hypotension [1].

In a prospective, randomized, controlled, and open pilot study evaluating the effects of continuous MB infusion on the hemodynamics and organic functions of human septic shock, Kirov et al. (2001) concluded that in human septic shock, MB with continuous infusion neutralizes myocardial depression, maintains oxygen transport, and reduces simultaneous adrenergic support. MB infusion does not appear to have significant adverse effects on selected organic function variables [2].

Ozal et al. (2005) prospectively studied whether preoperative administration of MB would prevent vasoplegic syndrome in these high-risk patients. Angiotensin-converting enzyme inhibitors, calcium channel blockers, and preoperative use of intravenous heparin are independent risk factors for vasoplegic syndrome after cardiac surgery. They did not include septic endocarditis as a risk factor. The results suggested that the preoperative administration of MB reduces the incidence and severity of vasoplegic syndrome in high-risk patients, thus ensuring adequate systemic vascular resistance in the operative and postoperative periods and shortening

P. R. Barbosa Evora et al., *Vasoplegic Endothelial Dysfunction*, https://doi.org/10.1007/978-3-030-74096-2_14

the intensive care unit and hospitalizations. Perhaps this report is the first suggestion of prophylactic use of MB before CPB [3].

The marked NO release, induced by the systemic inflammatory response associated with infective endocarditis (IE) and cardiopulmonary bypass (CPB), can result in hypotension refractory to catecholamine (vasoplegia) and increased need for transfusion due to platelet inhibition.

MB is an inducible NO-inhibiting drug. Cho et al. (2012) aimed to evaluate the effect of prophylactic administration of MB before CPB on the requirements of vasopressors and transfusions in patients with IE undergoing heart valve surgery (HVS). A total of 42 adult patients were randomly assigned to receive 2 mg.Kg^{-1} of MB (group MB, $n = 21$) or saline (control group, $n = 21$) for 20 minutes before the onset of CPB. The primary outcomes were comparisons of vasopressor needs assessed in series after weaning from CPB and hemodynamic parameters recorded in series before and after CPB. The secondary outcome was the comparison of transfusion requirements. Two patients in the control group received MB after weaning from CPB due to vasoplegia refractory to noradrenaline and vasopressin and, therefore, were excluded. There were no significant differences in vasopressor requirements and hemodynamic parameters between the two groups. The average number of packed red cell units transfused per transfused patient was significantly lower in the MB group. The number of patients transfused with fresh frozen plasma and platelet concentrate was lower in the MB group. The authors concluded that in patients with IE undergoing HVS, prophylactic administration of MB before CPB did not confer significant benefits in terms of vasopressor requirements and hemodynamic parameters but was associated with a substantial reduction in the need for transfusion [4].

We have used MB to treat refractory vasoplegias since 1994, and the specialized medical literature corroborates our experience. Most of our experience involved adults who had hypotension during cardiopulmonary bypass (CPB) or after the operation, a situation in which, like sepsis, NO plays a significant role. In this environment, two prospective and randomized studies came to definite conclusions about the efficacy of MB in the treatment or prevention of vasoplegic syndrome in patients undergoing cardiac surgery with the aid of CPB.

Taylor and Holtby (2005) presented a case of refractory hypotension in a child with native mitral valve endocarditis with brain complications in whom MB was less effective than previously described. Although Drs. Taylor and Holtby seemed disappointed with the effect of MB on blood pressure, we believe that their case had an impressive evolution despite its severity. We disagree that "the obvious clinical improvement using MB was not evident in this case" since most of the pharmacological support for circulation was needed for a short period [5].

In our opinion, the controversy over the use of MB to treat similar cases arises when someone uses the drug only as a kind of "last-minute vasopressor." Sometimes MB seems to work for this purpose, and sometimes it does not, perhaps because, unlike many vasopressors, MB does not act through a membrane receptor. We believe that the central action of MB is not exclusively the guanylyl cyclase blockage resulting in a reduction in guanosine 3'5'-cyclic monophosphate (cGMP). This blockage also improves the "cross talk" between the adenosine 3'5'-cyclic mono-phosphate (cAMP) and cGMP pathways, which facilitate the effect of cAMP-dependent vasopressors [4].

Reports in the medical literature, including the treatment of sepsis, prove that guanylyl cyclase blockage seems to improve the effect of vasopressors, decreasing the duration of pharmacological cardiovascular support. Another very advantageous but unproven effect of MB is its ability to reduce vascular permeability.

We operated in an emergency a young drug addict with native aortic valve endo-carditis. The patient received a bifold valve prosthesis (St Jude Medical, Inc, St Paul, MN). He came to the operating room using a high concentration of amines. A high dose of norepinephrine was necessary to maintain consistent blood pressure before and during cardiopulmonary bypass (CPB). After weaning from CPB, he presented hypotension and high cardiac output, low systemic vascular resistance, and pulmonary edema. Arterial oxygen saturation was below 80%, although he was being ventilated with 100% oxygen using positive end-expiratory pressure. We started the MB in a continuous infusion, in a remarkably similar way to that used by Dr. Taylor, followed by a bolus of 3 mg.Kg^{-1} (in 100 mL of 5% glucose in water) twice a day. Although mean arterial pressure did not increase even with norepineph-rine, cardiac output gradually decreased, and systemic vascular resistance increased. Also, the rapid resolution of pulmonary edema, resulting in higher arterial oxygen saturation, was surprising [5].

Protocol Proposal

These observations led us to propose a protocol with the use of MB in cases of emergency surgery in patients with vasoplegic syndrome: (1) 3 mg.Kg^{-1} bolus infu-sion right after anesthetic induction (perhaps even earlier); (2) infusion of 1 mg. Kg^{-1} (IV or in the oxygenator) if blood pressure maintenance is not possible due to high perfusion flow and high doses of norepinephrine; and (3) repeat the infusion in bolus (or continuous if the patient is stable) after CPB discontinuity.

Concluding Remarks

- Patients with an ongoing systemic inflammatory response because of infective endocarditis and those who need cardiopulmonary bypass (CPB) for emergency valve replacement may demonstrate resistant hypotension related to vasoplegia.
- It presents a spectrum of clinical presentation associated with a systemic inflam-matory response and endothelial nitric oxide release (NO).

- Hemodynamically, it is characterized by arterial vasodilation, high cardiac output despite myocardial depression, and decreased heart and peripheral vessels' sensitivity to sympathomimetic agents.
- These observations led us to propose a protocol using MB in emergency surgery cases in patients with vasoplegic syndrome: (1) 3 mg.Kg^{-1} bolus infusion right after anesthetic induction (perhaps even earlier); (2) infusion of 1 mg.Kg^{-1} (IV or in the oxygenator) if blood pressure maintenance is not possible due to high perfusion flow and high doses of norepinephrine; and (3) repeat the infusion in bolus (or continuous if the patient is stable) after CPB discontinuity.

References

1. Grayling M, Deakin CD. Methylene blue during cardiopulmonary bypass to treat refractory hypotension in septic endocarditis. J Thorac Cardiovasc Surg. 2003;125(2):426–7.
2. Kirov MY, Evgenov OV, Evgenov NV, Egorina EM, Sovershaev MA, Sveinbjornsson B, et al. Infusion of methylene blue in human septic shock: a pilot, randomized, controlled study. Crit Care Med. 2001;29(10):1860–7.
3. Ozal E, Kuralay E, Yildirim V, Kilic S, Bolcal C, Kucukarslan N, et al. Preoperative methylene blue administration in patients at high risk for vasoplegic syndrome during cardiac surgery. Ann Thorac Surg. 2005;79(5):1615–9.
4. Cho JS, Song JW, Na S, Moon JH, Kwak YL. Effect of a single bolus of methylene blue prophylaxis on vasopressor and transfusion requirement in infective endocarditis patients undergoing cardiac surgery. Korean J Anesthesiol. 2012;63(2):142–8.
5. Taylor K, Holtby H. Methylene blue revisited: management of hypotension in a pediatric patient with bacterial endocarditis. J Thorac Cardiovasc Surg. 2005;130(2):566.

Part IV
Endothelial Dysfunction in Specific Situations

Chapter 15
Vasoplegic Syndrome in Heart Surgery

One problem in describing vasoplegic syndrome (VS) is the lack of consistency in its definition. There is no clear definition, not even a single biomarker, including the determination of nitrite/nitrate (NOx) to characterize the syndrome. VS is a constellation of signs and symptoms: arterial hypotension, high cardiac index, low systemic vascular resistance, low filling pressure, and maintained arterial hypotension, despite the use of high doses of vasoconstrictor amines. This problem leads to a lack of definition of its incidence, varying from 0.21 to 13%. The most extensive series of prospective studies indicate a frequency of 8–12%. Mortality is high, ranging from 16% to 27%, and, therefore, has been the subject of several studies designed to improve the outcomes of these patients [1].

As a historical review, three facts individually mark the vasoplegic syndrome (VS) as a Brazilian contribution to cardiac surgery with cardiopulmonary bypass (CPB): (a) its description by Gomes et al., in 1994 [2]; (b) the proposal, also in 1994, that vasoplegia pathophysiology was guanosine 3′5′-cyclic monophosphate (cGMP)-dependent and methylene blue (MB) as its treatment; and (c) the documentation related to the first phase of this therapeutic efficiency proposed in patients undergoing cardiac surgery presented by Andrade et al. (1996) at the Congress of the Brazilian Society of Cardiovascular Surgery [3–5].

Although MB has been used for more than 20 years in the treatment of VS, few quality clinical studies can allow the procedure to become a protocol. Three studies, already mentioned in the epilogue, involving a more significant number of patients deserve special mention. (1) In 2003, Leyh et al. reported, in Germany, 54 cases of patients undergoing cardiac surgery, without endocarditis and treated with MB, with over 90% of patients responding to treatment [6]. (2) Levin et al., in Argentina, reported the incidence of 8.8% of VS in 638 patients [7]. The 56 patients with VS were randomly selected to receive MB or placebo, noting that there was no mortality in the MB group and that it was possible to stop the use of vasoconstrictors in a short time, with less consequent morbidity and mortality. In the placebo group, two deaths occurred, and the use of amines lasted an average of 48 hours, with a higher

P. R. Barbosa Evora et al., *Vasoplegic Endothelial Dysfunction*, https://doi.org/10.1007/978-3-030-74096-2_15

incidence of respiratory and kidney problems. (3) Regarding prevention, Ozal et al., in Turkey, showed in a prospective randomized study that MB was associated with a lower incidence of vasoplegia and use of amines [8]. The situation of hemodynamic instability after cardiac surgery has been described as a post-perfusion syndrome, vasoplegic syndrome, and low peripheral vascular resistance syndrome, all of which can be included in the general terminology of systemic inflammatory response syndrome (SIRS). This situation has been responsible for deaths in cardiac surgery, often in cases whose surgical indication is not associated with high risk, which leads to an extremely dramatic situation. It is triggered, at least in part, by cardiopulmonary bypass, and contributes substantially to morbidity (e.g., myocardial depression) and mortality in patients undergoing cardiac surgery.

The primary mechanism of this inflammatory response is related to the complement cascade, the activation of blood cells, the cytokines release, and the nitric oxide (NO) synthesis induction. The relative importance of each factor, however, is still a matter of debate.

Risk stratification systems based on cytokine measurements demonstrate early inflammatory response detection in 2–10% of all patients, which is associated with a worsening prognosis. This text intends to review these experimental, pathophysiological, clinical, and therapeutic aspects, highlighting the role of MB, which, in the authors' experience, has been a lifesaving measure.

Pathophysiology

The pathophysiology of vasoplegia after cardiopulmonary bypass is multifactorial, with no final consensus on its real mechanism. For didactic purposes, emphasis will be given to three aspects, which are the most mentioned in clinical and laboratory studies on the subject: (a) the systemic inflammatory reaction; (b) the effects of protamine; and (c) a new mechanism recently related to the impairment of vasopressin receptors.

Systemic Inflammatory Reaction

The modern era of cardiac surgery began when the technique for the cardiopulmonary bypass was introduced in the early 1950s. Cardiopulmonary bypass (CPB) is indispensable for most cardiac surgeries, but an undesirable inflammatory reaction occurs because of its use. In an attempt to understand the pathophysiology of vasoplegic syndrome, several pathogenic hypotheses have been raised, including (a) bacterial and viral infections; (b) immunological reactions related to anti myocardial antibodies; and (c) anaphylactoid reactions associated with anesthetics, protamine, heparin, and the extracorporeal circulation circuit itself [9].

Many factors during CPB, dependent on its material (blood exposure to non-physiological surfaces and conditions) or independent of its material (surgical trauma, ischemia-reperfusion of the organs, changes in body temperature, and endotoxin release), have been well documented as inducing a complex inflammatory response. These factors include complement system activation, cytokine release, leukocyte activation, and adhesion molecule expression, in addition to the production of various substances, such as oxygen free radicals, arachidonic acid metabolites, platelet activation factor, NO, and endothelin. This inflammatory cascade can contribute to the development of postoperative complications, including respiratory failure, renal dysfunction, hemorrhagic disorders, neurological dysfunction, changes in liver function, and, ultimately, multiple organ failure. More recently, it has been observed that this anti-inflammatory response can begin during and after cardiopulmonary bypass. This complex chain of events has strong similarities to sepsis. Regarding the extracorporeal circulation circuit, it should be noted that its incidence is higher with the use of bubble oxygenators compared to membrane oxygenators [9].

The pathophysiology remains unclear, and a logical sequence of events can be outlined: pro-inflammatory and/or inflammatory stimulus. As a consequence there is an activation of the complement system, the release of various cytokines (interleukins, tumor necrosis factor, platelet activation factor, etc.), activation of the inducible form of nitric oxide synthase (iNOS), production of NO, and activation of guanylate cyclase with increased cGMP that leads to refractory vasoplegia even with the use of high doses of adrenergic amines.

There is also a tendency to diffuse bleeding due to NO antiplatelet activities. The schematic representation of this inflammatory response can be seen in Fig. 15.1.

Regarding the participation of NO, it is curious to note that a clinical study measuring nitrates in the urine and blood of patients undergoing cardiac surgery with cardiopulmonary bypass has not shown a correlation between endogenous NO and low systemic vascular resistance.

Regarding the mechanisms involved, individually, some data deserve to be highlighted [10]:

1. The clinical relevance of complement activation alone is still uncertain. Several studies have related postoperative morbidity with complement activation.

Fig. 15.1 Vasoplegic syndrome in cardiac surgery

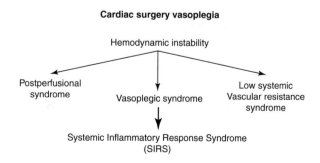

2. The prevention of neutrophil adhesion can bring practical benefits, but these benefits can be associated with an increased risk of infection.
3. Leukocyte activation can release large amounts of oxygen free radicals, including the superoxide anion, hydrogen peroxide, the hydroxyl radical, and oxygen itself. These radicals act on lipid membranes, increasing permeability, which can compromise cardiac and pulmonary functions.
4. The products of arachidonic acid metabolism (prostaglandins, thromboxane A2, and leukotrienes) can be counterbalanced by the joint production of vasodilating prostaglandins, such as prostacyclin (PGI-2). Leukotrienes may be responsible for increasing capillary permeability.
5. Endotoxin levels may increase during and after cardiopulmonary bypass. The sources of endotoxins are as varied as possible; however, the most crucial font is the intestines. Splanchnic vasoconstriction during cardiopulmonary bypass can lead to ischemia and increased permeability of the intestinal loops, with the endotoxins released into the bloodstream. Endotoxin levels are related to initial vasoconstriction, aortic clamping time, and hypo-oncotic state during cardiopulmonary bypass.
6. Cytokine release can be stimulated by several factors, including ischemia-reperfusion, complement activation, endotoxin release, and the effect of other cytokines.
7. The platelet activation factor plays an essential role in the myocardial ischemia-reperfusion injury and may also have deleterious hemodynamic effects during cardiopulmonary bypass.
8. The excessive NO production by the iNOS expression may be the final consequence of these multiple mechanisms, being the primary cause of the vasoplegic syndrome.
9. There may be an increase in endothelin levels during cardiopulmonary bypass during the surgical treatment of congenital heart disease, heart valve disease, and myocardial revascularization. Its role, however, is not very clear in the pathophysiology of vasoplegia after cardiopulmonary bypass. Anyway, if vasoplegia is a consequence of a significant NO release, its opposing vasoconstrictor effect is not manifested.
10. There is a current tendency to change the paradigm that the inflammatory reaction associated with VS would be caused by the exposure of blood to the non-endothelial surface of CPB after it was found that the inflammatory response is present in patients operated without CPB. The changing trend is associated with the concept that, more than contact with the CPB circuit, the communication of blood with the surgical wound would be the main responsible for the inflammatory phenomenon.

Reactions Caused by Protamine

Horrow classified the results caused by protamine in three different categories:

(a) Systemic hypotension as a common reaction
(b) Anaphylactoid responses
(c) Catastrophic pulmonary hypertension

The precise mechanism that explains protamine-induced hypotension is not fully understood. It appears that its effect on reducing peripheral vascular resistance plays a more important role than its impact on cardiac function. With constant monitoring of cardiac output, systemic blood pressure, and ventricular pressures of patients during protamine infusion after extracorporeal circulation, it was found that protamine causes a significant reduction in peripheral vascular resistance. This hypotension occurs when the increase in cardiac output is insufficient to compensate for decreased peripheral resistance.

Four experimental trials conducted at the Mayo Clinic (Rochester, MN, United States) studied the intrinsic mechanism of vasodilation caused by protamine, demonstrating that the endothelium and nitric oxide (NO) play an important role.

The first study showed that NO is released in vitro by the systemic circulation and the coronary circulation after protamine infusion. The main results of this study were (a) protamine induces the NO release and (b) endothelium-dependent vasodilation caused by protamine is not affected by heparin and indomethacin. Thus, it was concluded that protamine decreases vascular tone, inducing the release of NO. Since indomethacin does not affect vasodilation, prostacyclin may not be involved as a mediator.

The second study demonstrated that the pulmonary circulation is hugely affected by the action of protamine in the endothelial function, releasing NO; this release can be inhibited by blocking NO synthesis with N^G-monomethyl-L-arginine (L-NMMA), but not by blocking prostacyclin with indomethacin. Unlike what happens in the systemic and coronary circulation, heparin prevents endothelium-dependent vasodilation, which only manifests itself with higher doses of protamine. The third study demonstrated in vivo that L-NMMA (blocking NO synthesis) and MB (blocking guanylate cyclase) antagonized the vasodilator effects of protamine.

Finally, a fourth study demonstrated endothelium-dependent vasodilation in microcirculation vessels through a hyperpolarization mechanism, maybe with the likely participation of an unknown endothelium-derived hyperpolarizing factor.

From a cardiocirculatory point of view, the state of shock can be classified into three groups: (1) primary or secondary myocardial failure, (2) acute loss of volume or vascular obstruction, and (3) alteration of vascular capacitance. Although this classification is useful for academic discussions, clinical presentations are more involved with different pathophysiological mechanisms present in the same patient (e.g., septic shock associated with hypovolemia and myocardial depression). The capacitance changes correspond to the circulatory shock called distributive shock, where the vasoplegic syndrome in cardiac surgery fits, described by Gomes et al.

(1994), which later confirmed to be a manifestation of the systemic inflammatory response syndrome (SIRS) (Fig. 15.1) [2].

This syndrome has its pathophysiology with the same characteristics as sepsis, that is, vasoplegia, a hyperdynamic state with high cardiac output and resistance to the use of high concentrations of catecholamines.

Clinical Aspects

The vasoplegic syndrome is clinically characterized by tachycardia, oliguria, good peripheral perfusion, significant arterial hypotension with inadequate response to the use of high doses of catecholamines, and a notable tendency to diffuse bleeding (Table 15.1). In nonrandomized observations, an amazing situation of prolonged hypotension is often observed in patients undergoing revascularization of multiple coronary arteries, without episodes of ischemia and/or myocardial infarction, observable by monitoring the electrocardiogram at the bedside. The presence of myocardial failure is not observed by itself. It is noted, as already mentioned, the presence of vasodilation with hypotension refractory to catecholamines and, in some cases, the presence of significant tachycardia.

In our daily practice, vasoplegia has been of interest for about 10 years. In search of a cause-effect relationship, several aspects were considered:

1. Most cases occurred during or after cardiopulmonary bypass.
2. In the past, there have been several cases associated with the use of curare allopherine during anesthetic induction.
3. Some cases, more attenuated, occurred during anesthetic induction using a standardized technique with etomidate, fentanyl, Pavulon, and diazepine.
4. Some cases were associated with the use of protamine.
5. In some cases, that vasodilation apparently occurred after the use of heparin.
6. Vasoplegic syndrome was observed in noncardiac surgeries.
7. There is the impression that the cases arise in outbreaks.
8. There is no relationship with the type of surgical heart disease.
9. Many patients have diabetes.
10. Several patients had previously used the calcium antagonist diltiazem.

These observations can be added to the possible effects of angiotensin-converting enzyme inhibitors, angiotensin II inhibitors, and even the use of amiodarone.

Table 15.1 Clinical aspects of vasoplegic syndrome

The Vasoplegic syndrome is clinically characterized by:
Tachycardia
Good peripheral perfusion
Significant arterial hypotension with inadequate response to the use of high doses of catecholamines
Notable tendency to diffuse bleeding

In a letter to the editor of *The Journal of Thoracic and Cardiovascular Surgery*, Poullis draws attention to a series of medications that, used preoperatively, may in some way be associated with vasoplegias in cardiac surgery. For example, angiotensin II decreases the vasopressin release by the neurohypophysis. Thus, inhibitors of this polypeptide as losartan may be associated with the distributive shock. Most patients have no complications related to angiotensin-converting enzyme inhibitors, even if suspended on the morning of the surgery. Therefore, further observations are necessary to attribute some clinical importance to this type of medication as part of the pathophysiology of vasoplegia in cardiac surgery. Its common association with amiodarone could be related to mechanisms of vasodilation, e.g., alpha and beta blocks associated with inhibition of the angiotensin-converting enzyme, decreased angiotensin II, and reduced vasopressin release. It is worth mentioning the use of nicorandil, a medication that, by opening potassium channels, may be associated with a decrease in systemic vascular resistance, requiring greater use of vasoconstrictors in cardiac surgery. Finally, it is necessary to report that patients on long-term use of angiotensin-converting enzyme inhibitors before cardiac surgery generally need more catecholamines in the perioperative period and those who do not receive the drug again in the postoperative period face a risk of impairment of microcirculation, configuring an additional reason for the onset of vasoplegic syndrome.

Since vasoplegia can be detected before, during, and after cardiopulmonary bypass, the terminology "post-perfusion vasoplegia" is questioned, being the most widespread problem. This terminology was avoided in this text since the phenomenon can be observed in patients undergoing myocardial revascularization without extracorporeal circulation or even in noncardiac surgeries. In some patients, the onset of symptoms may be delayed due to compensatory mechanisms such as increased cardiac output and the release of catecholamines. In our daily medical practice, we have already identified some situations in which the MB use may or may not be useful [11].

Situation 1 A patient who underwent cardiac surgery with cardiopulmonary bypass showed signs of vasodilation, tachycardia, hypotension refractory to high doses of catecholamines, and increased blood lactate. The situation was reversed using MB and metoprolol. This situation can occur before, during, and in the immediate postoperative period. When it occurs during cardiopulmonary bypass, hypotension is also refractory to increased blood flow. The systemic inflammatory response is considered "vasoplegic syndrome."

Situation 2 A patient that underwent surgery with cardiopulmonary bypass. After cardiopulmonary bypass discontinuation and cannula removal, when proceeding with the neutralization of heparin with protamine, the patient presented severe hypotension resistant to amine bolus, followed by cardiac arrest. Upon returning to cardiopulmonary bypass, blood pressure remained irresponsive to high blood flows and high doses of amines. The heart started beating with an electrocardiogram without significant changes except for an elevated heart rate. The situation was reversed using MB and metoprolol.

Situation 3 A septuagenarian, diabetic, hypertensive, smoker patient, who underwent technically challenging myocardial revascularization. In the postoperative unit, he had significant bleeding, requiring surgical revision. On the 7th day, he started to experience chills, hypothermia, hypotension, and tachycardia. With an infectious blood count, eliminating purulent secretion through sternotomy, he was again taken to the operating room, where the presence of severe mediastinitis was found. The patient had hypotension with tachycardia several times, which were controlled using MB and metoprolol. The patient died after 5 days.

Situation 4 A young patient who underwent valve surgery with cardiopulmonary bypass, developed without complications. In the preoperative period, he had an inevitable increase in nitrogen compounds and a history of renal colic. In the infirmary, he began to manifest low back pain and a marked fall in diuresis. After an ultrasound showing a single "horseshoe" kidney, the urologist opted for excretory urography with radiated contrast, during which there was a severe anaphylactic reaction with hypotension, bradycardia, and facial angioedema, with no response to adrenaline, corticosteroids, and volumetric expansion. The situation was reversed with the use of MB.

Situation 5 A patient undergoing emergency surgery for aortic dissection. For correction, it was necessary to use deep hypothermia. After the rewarming phase, with the release of the aortic clamping, the heartbeat recovered spontaneously. However, it showed refractory hypotension at any measure, and extracorporeal circulation was not possible. The use of MB in cardiopulmonary bypass did not alter blood pressure in any way, characterizing a situation different from the previous ones.

Hemodynamic Aspects

Although most shock states are associated with decreased cardiac output, a different situation occurs in cases of shocks due to reduced vascular capacitance where vasoplegia is associated with increased cardiac output, configuring a hyperdynamic situation with severe hypotension resistant to high doses of catecholamines (Table 15.2).

It is essential to report that even in this situation, myocardial depression can occur with low ejection fractions and biventricular dilation [11].

The poor prognosis seems to be better correlated with low vascular resistance, leading to the conclusion that vasoplegia is the determining prognostic factor. Thus,

Table 15.2 Hemodynamic traits of the vasoplegic syndrome

Hemodynamic profile
Hypotension
Low filling pressures
Normal or high cardiac index
Low peripheral vascular resistance
Need for high doses of vasopressors

the paracrine endothelial control of vascular capacitance, mainly due to the action of NO, becomes an essential factor for clinical and experimental investigations in the search for new pathophysiological and therapeutic knowledge that can contribute to the treatment and prognosis of vasoplegia. It should be noted that endothelial dysfunction is associated with all types of shock.

Therapeutic Aspects

The approach includes (1) the use of corticosteroids to inhibit the inflammatory reaction and block the iNOS action; (2) use of norepinephrine, as it is an amine that does not promote an increase in heart rate, and may even decrease it; (3) use of MB (2 mg.Kg^{-1} of weight in intravenous bolus or half the bolus dose, followed by continuous infusion of additional dosages); and (4) use of injectable metoprolol (5 mg) to reverse the situation of downregulation of beta-receptors, which is a consequence of tachycardia and the use of amines. Because of this phenomenon, fewer beta receptors are available for effective action of beta-adrenergic drugs, with tachyphylaxis occurring [10].

Regarding the treatment regimen with MB, there is still no therapeutic protocol scheme. The dosage used to treat methemoglobinemia and sepsis (2 mg.Kg^{-1} IV bolus) has been adopted. As its plasma concentration decreases dramatically during the first 40 minutes of bolus infusion, we have been maintaining the same dose in continuous infusion for the next hour. There are personal reports of its use at up to 7 mg.Kg^{-1}, without side effects. Since the lethal dose, determined in goats, is 40 mg. Kg^{-1}, we believe that, in extreme cases, the use of a total dosage of up to 10 mg.Kg^{-1} is safe.

It should be noted that this is an assumption and cannot be considered a therapeutic principle. There is at least one report, at a dose of 10 mg.Kg^{-1}, without complications and with clinical improvement of patients and systemic vascular resistance, lactate, and norepinephrine.

Two technical aspects must be highlighted: the MB injection interferes with pulse oximetry, giving the false impression of arterial unsaturation, this effect being temporary, and the false drop in lactate levels. In reality, the decrease in the measured lactate occurs by reaction with MB, giving the wrong impression of better adequacy of tissue perfusion.

It is imperative to avoid excess fluid replacement, the main objective is to reverse vasoplegia with vasoconstrictors and MB. As hypotension is refractory to the use of amines, the use of MB has been lifesaving. The option to use arginine vasopressin is quite attractive, but there are still no clinical experiments with this drug, although some experimental trials have been carried out.

The action of NO depends on the activation of the cGMP system. Still, in addition to this vital mechanism of significant importance, attention has also been directed to the adenosine $3'5'$-cyclic monophosphate (cAMP) system, which is why the injectable beta-blocker (metoprolol) is being used, almost as a routine, in cases where the patient is very tachycardic.

Another logical approach would be to inhibit NO synthesis with the use of specific inhibitors, such as N^G-Nitro-L-Arginine Methyl Ester (L-NAME) and L-NMMA. This approach is open to criticism and involves ethical problems related to the use of new therapies, in addition to blocking not only the inducible form of nitric oxide synthase (iNOS) but also the physiological form of this enzyme (cNOS). The use of specific iNOS inhibition, for example, with aminoguanidine, remains in the logical and speculative territories. The use of MB would not have these problems since it does not block the synthesis of NO and because it is a medication widely used in other clinical conditions. Its lethal dose is 40 mg.Kg^{-1}, which is far from those used in the treatment of post-perfusion systemic inflammatory response syndrome. The action of MB implies the inhibition of guanylate cyclase, preventing the elevation of cGMP and, consequently, avoiding the endothelium-dependent relaxation mediated by NO.

Other Possible Therapeutic Strategies

Corticosteroids have been used in cardiac surgery for more than 30 years. Its use is attributed to a series of effects: (1) improvement of hemodynamic conditions; (2) less vasoconstriction with improved tissue perfusion; (3) cellular effects, such as the stabilization of the lysosome membrane; (4) inhibition of phospholipase A2 activation, with stabilization of lipid cell membranes; (5) anti-inflammatory activity, with less release of cytokines and inhibition of complement activation; and (6) selective inhibition of iNOS, demonstrated experimentally by the action of dexamethasone. Although its use has an experimental and logical basis, numerous studies have failed to prove its real effectiveness [10].

Some studies attempt to attribute anti-inflammatory activity to aprotinin, in situations of ischemia-reperfusion and in association with the use of oxygenators with heparinized surfaces, but the controversial aspects regarding its real effectiveness do not justify its routine use. Likewise, the use of antioxidants in the preoperative period, the use of oxygenators with a heparinized surface, and leukocyte depletion are also speculative matters. The techniques of ultrafiltration and "cell savers" may perhaps be considered necessary, as they are used almost as a routine in American services, where one has the impression that vasoplegic shock is not a problem as marked as in our environment. The removal of pro-inflammatory substances and the decrease in the contact of white blood cells with the extracorporeal circulation circuit are certainly useful functions of these two techniques [10].

Conclusion

Finally, MB is an option for the treatment of VS in cases of failure of the first-line treatment (careful volume adjustment and use of amines). The early use of MB can block the progression of falling systemic vascular resistance in patients responsive to norepinephrine and mitigate the need for a prolonged use of vasoconstrictors.

However, regimes and protocols need to be clearly defined for their routine use. Whether MB can be a first-line treatment in patients with vasoplegia is a matter of debate, and there is still no evidence to support this.

Evidence-based studies point to the need for more scientific evidence to define the role of MB in the treatment of VS refractory to the use of amines. One of these studies, of our authorship, was assisted by a Scottish researcher specialized in evidence-based medicine. We think that the experimental evidence is conclusive, requiring new extensive multicenter studies, adopting the principles of the reviews of Levin (Argentina) and Ozal (Turkey) [7, 8].

From the historical analysis, it is clear that the MB use, specifically in VS associated with cardiac surgery, is a Brazilian contribution. Its use in sepsis is already established without the use of extensive multicenter studies confirming the inflammatory phenomenon as the primary mechanism involved. Assigning a possible role to "vasopressin deficiency" as the most important mechanism of VS is, at the very least, reckless. Although there are no definitive multicentric studies, and despite all the "snags," the MB used in the treatment of VS in cardiac surgery is currently the best, safest, and most inexpensive option, being a Brazilian contribution to cardiac surgery.

Concluding Remarks

- Vasoplegic syndrome (VS) is a constellation of signs and symptoms: arterial hypotension, high cardiac index, low systemic vascular resistance, low filling pressure, and maintained arterial hypotension, despite the use of high doses of vasoconstrictor amines.
- The situation of hemodynamic instability after cardiac surgery has been described as post-perfusion syndrome, vasoplegic syndrome, and low peripheral vascular resistance syndrome, all of which can be included in the general terminology of systemic inflammatory response syndrome (SIRS).
- There is strong evidence that methylene blue (MB), a guanylate cyclase inhibitor, is an excellent therapeutic option for the treatment of vasoplegic syndrome (VS) in cardiac surgery. Our clinical and laboratory experience, accumulated over a period of 20 years, established some classic concepts about the use of MB in this condition.
- Heparin and ACE inhibitors are considered risk factors.
- In the recommended doses, MB is a safe drug (the lethal dose is 40 mg.Kg^{-1}).
- MB does not cause endothelial dysfunction.
- The effect of MB appears only in the case of nitric oxide (NO) overregulation.
- MB is not a vasoconstrictor; by blocking the guanosine 3′5′-cyclic monophosphate (cGMP) system, it "releases" the adenosine 3′5′-cyclic monophosphate(cAMP) system, facilitating the vasoconstrictor effect of norepinephrine.
- The most used dosage is 2 mg.Kg^{-1} in intravenous bolus, followed by continuous infusion, as the plasma concentration declines sharply in the first 40 minutes.

- There is a possible "window of opportunity" for MB effectiveness.
- Although there are no definitive multicenter studies, the use of MB in the treatment of VS in cardiac surgery is currently the best, safest, and cheapest option, being a Brazilian contribution.

References

1. Gomes WJ, Evora PR. Vasoplegic syndrome after off-pump coronary artery bypass surgery: a rising threat. Eur J Cardiothorac Surg. 2009;35(6):1116–7.
2. Gomes WJ, Carvalho AC, Palma JH, Goncalves I Jr, Buffolo E. Vasoplegic syndrome: a new dilemma. J Thorac Cardiovasc Surg. 1994;107(3):942–3.
3. Andrade JCS, Batista Filho ML, Evora PRB, Tavares JR, Buffolo E, Ribeiro EE, et al. Utilização do azul de metileno no tratamento da síndrome vasoplégica após cirurgia cardíaca. Rev Bras Cir Cardiovasc. 1996;11(2):107–14.
4. Evora PR, Ribeiro PJ, de Andrade JC. Methylene blue administration in SIRS after cardiac operations. Ann Thorac Surg. 1997;63(4):1212–3.
5. Evora PR. Should methylene blue be the drug of choice to treat vasoplegias caused by cardiopulmonary bypass and anaphylactic shock? J Thorac Cardiovasc Surg. 2000;119(3):632–4.
6. Leyh RG, Kofidis T, Struber M, Fischer S, Knobloch K, Wachsmann B, et al. Methylene blue: the drug of choice for catecholamine-refractory vasoplegia after cardiopulmonary bypass? J Thorac Cardiovasc Surg. 2003;125(6):1426–31.
7. Levin RL, Degrange MA, Bruno GF, Del Mazo CD, Taborda DJ, Griotti JJ, et al. Methylene blue reduces mortality and morbidity in vasoplegic patients after cardiac surgery. Ann Thorac Surg. 2004;77(2):496–9.
8. Ozal E, Kuralay E, Yildirim V, Kilic S, Bolcal C, Kucukarslan N, et al. Preoperative methylene blue administration in patients at high risk for vasoplegic syndrome during cardiac surgery. Ann Thorac Surg. 2005;79(5):1615–9.
9. Mota AL, Rodrigues AJ, Evora PR. [Adult cardiopulmonary bypass in the twentieth century: science, art or empiricism?]. Rev Bras Cir Cardiovasc. 2008;23(1):78–92.
10. Evora PR, Bottura C, Arcencio L, Albuquerque AA, Evora PM, Rodrigues AJ. Key points for curbing cardiopulmonary bypass inflammation. Acta Cir Bras. 2016;31 Suppl 1:45–52.
11. Luciano PM, Araujo WF, Rodrigues AJ, Evora PRB. Vasoplegic syndrome in cardiac surgery. In: Moock M, Filho AB, editors. Intensive care - training for the specialist title test of the Brazilian Association of Intensive Care Medicine. 1. Barueri/SP: Manole Ltda; 2008. p. 412–25.

Chapter 16
Vasoplegic Endothelial Dysfunction in Orthotopic Liver Transplantation

Since the experience with methylene blue (MB) is more considerable in cases of liver transplantation, the concepts presented in this chapter will be more based on this type of transplant.

The nitric oxide/guanosine 3′5′-cyclic monophosphate (NO/cGMP) pathway should have a significant influence on the hemodynamic changes that occur in this clinical setting. Classically, the post-reperfusion syndrome is characterized by hypotension and low vascular resistance after blood flow restoration, when cGMP and NO are increased by positive regulation induced by nitric oxide synthase (NOS). The increase in the level of cytokines and endotoxins, resulting in a systemic inflammatory response, is the mediator of the positive NOS regulation. The production of large NO amounts causes vasodilation and oxidative stress. These mechanisms in various types of transplants, such as the liver, heart, lungs, and kidney, are the critical point for grafts. Also, it is essential that, in the end, the significant relationship between graft dysfunction or rejection and ischemia-reperfusion injury is known, which is linked to the inflammatory response and activation of the NO/cGMP pathway (Fig. 16.1). Therefore, this review aims to study the NO/cGMP pathway in solid organ transplants. Finally, we asked whether the NO/cGMP pathway is underestimated by doctors, suggesting that inhibition by MB is useful, safe, and lifesaving in vasoplegia of resistant amines caused by reperfusion of organ grafts [1].

The massive NO production by the inducible isoform of nitric oxide synthase (iNOS) is considered responsible for deep vasodilation and myocardial dysfunction in septic shock. The number of liver procedures is increasing worldwide; however, the NO role in cirrhosis risk score (CRS) in liver transplantation is still unknown. The ischemia and reperfusion syndrome observed during liver transplant surgery can manifest itself as a vasoplegic state that often requires vasopressor support to maintain stable hemodynamics. Occasionally, conventional treatment for this vasoplegic syndrome (VS) (e.g., phenylephrine, norepinephrine, and vasopressin) is not sufficient to restore adequate systemic vascular resistance (SVR) and systemic pressure support. These data, although incipient, motivated inclusion in this chapter [1].

P. R. Barbosa Evora et al., *Vasoplegic Endothelial Dysfunction*, https://doi.org/10.1007/978-3-030-74096-2_16

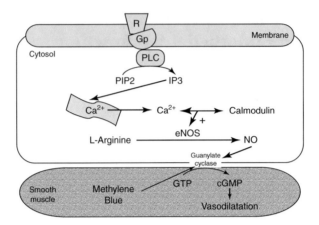

Fig. 16.1 The classical endothelial NO launch pathway requires: (1) signal transduction from a cell receptor-mediated via G proteins (Gp); (2) phospholipase C (PLC) activation and manufacturing of inositol triphosphate (IP3) from phosphatidylinositol 4,5-biphosphate (PIP2) and cytosolic Ca^{2+} release; (3) the constitutive endothelial nitric oxide synthase (eNOS) is activated by means of complicated Ca^{2+}/calmodulin and produces NO from its substrate L-arginine; (4) NO stimulates guanylate cyclase in adjoining easy muscle cells, which causes an extend in guanosine 3'5'-cyclic monophosphate (cGMP) that is the final stimulus that motives vasorelaxation; and (5) methylene blue inhibits the recreation of guanylate cyclase, lowering the cGMP production and less vascular clean muscle rest. (Adapted from Evora and Simon. Ann Allergy Asthma Immunol. 2007;99:306–13)

The Monophosphatic Changes of Cyclic Guanosine After Reperfusion Organ Transplantation

The mechanism of hemodynamic instability during organ transplantation is undoubtedly multifactorial. Although risk factors may be associated with the characteristics of organ receptors, such as reduced levels of vasopressin or diastolic dysfunction of the left ventricle, or related to ischemia time or the surgical technique, it is reasonable to assume that dysregulation of NO production leads to increased cGMP synthesis and an organic vasodilation stage probably contributes to vasoplegic syndrome. For example, the activation of cGMP production in patients with terminal liver disease has been associated with hemodynamic instability during liver transplantation.

Bezinover et al. (2013) confirmed that cGMP is one of the factors that contribute to intraoperative hypotension during liver transplantation. These authors also demonstrated that preoperative cGMP levels might have a possible prognostic value, suggesting the positive predictive value of preoperative cGMP levels in intraoperative hemodynamic instability. The excessive generation of NO derived from iNOS during liver reperfusion can result in circulatory shock. There is also evidence that the vasoplegia may be due to independent pathways of NO/cGMP because the soluble guanylate cyclase (sGC) can be activated for interleukins or oxygen free radicals in the absence of NO [2].

These conclusions typify the pivotal cGMP role in solid organ transplantation; the pathway is presented in Fig. 16.1.

Ischemia-Reperfusion Syndrome (IRS)

Reperfusion is an inevitable result of any organ subjected to ischemia for therapeutic purposes, such as transplantation or cardiac surgery, resulting in severe cell damage that contributes to the morbidity and mortality associated with the operation. The cell injury that occurs after the start of reperfusion is a consequence of the interaction of oxidative stress, local and systemic inflammatory response, and metabolic disorders, such as acidosis [3].

Ischemia-reperfusion syndrome (IRS) resulting in hypotension and increased postoperative transaminases is observed in most patients undergoing liver transplantation, and, in severe cases, this can lead to graft failure and death. Ischemia in the transplanted liver results in the degradation of adenosine triphosphate to hypoxanthine and the conversion of xanthine dehydrogenase to xanthine oxidase. During reperfusion, xanthine oxidase catalyzes the reaction between hypoxanthine and oxygen to produce xanthine and superoxide radicals and the production of oxygen free radicals, such as hydroxyl radicals, and hypochlorous acid. These reactive oxygen species (ROS) disrupt cell membranes and activate monocytes and neutrophils with the ROS mediators. After graft reperfusion, there is a decrease in mean arterial pressure (MAP) and systemic vascular resistance (SVR) and an increase in the cardiac index (CI), which often persists for 1–2 hours. Some patients have reduced myocardial contractility. The precise mechanisms underlying these hemodynamic responses are not yet fully understood. Thus, the ischemia-reperfusion syndrome (IRS) is characterized by persistent hypotension, with low systemic vascular resistance. The consequent syndrome is defined as a 30% decrease in MAP and occurs within 5 minutes of graft reperfusion, lasting at least 1 minute. Hypotension associated with low SVR can persist for an hour or more. The severity of the IRS is probably the result of both and contributes to impaired liver function in the postoperative period and primary graft failure (Fig. 16.2) [4].

Guanylate Cyclase Inhibition in Vasoplegia After Orthotopic Hepatic Transplantation

Methylene blue (MB) dye has been used as a vasopressor in sepsis and acute liver failure. When these conditions are associated with low MAP, an intravenous bolus of MB increases MAP by an increase in SVR and, in some cases, the cardiac index (CI). Sepsis and IRS show hemodynamic and biochemical similarities, including patterns of increased pro-inflammatory cytokines. In sepsis, these changes are

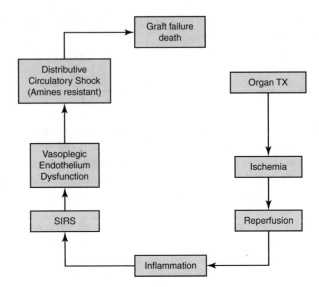

Fig. 16.2 Graft dysfunction or rejection and ischemia-reperfusion damage that is linked to inflammatory response and NO/cGMP pathway activation

associated with excess NO. MB acts reducing the NO action by inhibiting guanylate cyclase, the NO target enzyme.

In many previous studies, MB at doses of 1–3 mg.Kg^{-1} caused hemodynamic improvement in sepsis and acute liver failure. The dosage of 1.5–3 mg.Kg^{-1} is the most used, as proposed by the British National Formulary. Most clinical studies on sepsis have failed to demonstrate a change in hepatic failure (HF). However, in clinical practice, in the situation of the hyperdynamic state, an increase in MAP and SVR is observed with better hepatic function adequacy at lower levels. Otherwise, in in vitro experiments using tissues from animals treated with endotoxin, MB caused an increase in myocardial contractility in the left ventricle. Therefore, the changes observed in SVR and cardiac output may depend on the clinical situation.

Several modes of action of MB have been postulated. Different mechanisms can predominate in various clinical situations. The MB has proven to have blocking properties by inhibition of guanylate cyclase and possibly by inhibition of NOS. It also acts as an antioxidant and pro-oxidant, inhibits prostacyclin synthesis, and accelerates the reducing processes in the cell.

Guanylate Cyclase Inhibition in Hepatic Cirrhosis

Some authors have reported an increase in nitrite levels in patients with cirrhosis but not in non-cirrhotic patients. Post hoc analysis based on these reports showed that nitrite levels were significantly increased in patients with cirrhosis. There was a decrease in the level of nitrite after using MB in the cirrhosis group, but not in the non-cirrhotic group suggesting that different pathways for NO production could be involved in cirrhotic and non-cirrhotic patients.

Clinical Experience with Methylene Blue in Orthotopic Transplantation

In the last 25 years, the literature describes many clinical cases that use MB in the therapeutic approach of shock and vasoplegia refractory to conventional vasopressor therapy. For this reason, MB has been advocated to reverse the effects of vasodilatory shock. However, there is no widespread acceptance of its use in this clinical circumstance.

The mechanism of action of MB is based on the direct inhibition of sGC by oxidation of the ferrous iron bound to the enzyme. MB also interacts with sGC by binding to the iron heme complex. Consequently, it avoids the increase in cGMP and vascular relaxation mediated by NO, a fact closely linked to the pathophysiology of shock. Another effect of MB is its action as a selective iNOS inhibitor, reducing the overall NO production and preventing the increase in radical peroxynitrite and peroxynitrous acid. In addition to its effect on sGC and iNOS, MB inhibits the production of reactive oxygen species, acting as an alternative electron receptor for xanthine oxidase, competing with molecular oxygen for electron transfer. Electrons are transferred to MB from the iron-sulfur center of xanthine oxidase, preventing the conversion of molecular oxygen into superoxide. Therefore, MB contributes to mitigating the reperfusion injury caused by free radicals, a phenomenon inherent in any transplanted organ. Finally, sGC can be subtracted from interleukins and oxygen-free radicals, explaining why MB can improve vasoplegia, even in the absence of increased NO production.

The same questions, answers, doubts, and certainties are pertinent here. We reevaluated these concepts established in 20 years, with an emphasis on the last 5 years:

1. The recommended doses are safe (the lethal dose is 40 mg.Kg^{-1}).
2. Intravenous MB does not cause endothelial dysfunction.
3. The effect of intravenous MB appears in cases of positive NO regulation.
4. MB is not a vasoconstrictor.
5. The MB can act through this "cross talk" mechanism.
6. The most used dosage is 2 mg.Kg^{-1} in an intravenous bolus, followed by the same dosage for continuous infusion, as plasma concentrations fall sharply in the first 40 minutes.
7. There are no definitive multicenter studies involving MB, and, currently, it is the best or perhaps the safest and cheapest option.
8. For the effectiveness of MB, there is a possible "window of opportunity" [5].

The hemodynamic and metabolic effects of MB cannot be seen due to this "window of opportunity". In the first 8 hours of the systemic inflammatory reaction, there is an increase in the activity of NOS and an increase in sGC regulation. In the next 8 hours, there is a lack of sGC expression and negative NOS control. In the third 8-hour window, there is a positive regulation of guanylate cyclase (GC) and NOS.

We have emphasized two practical aspects: (1) disclosure in the use of MB, without considering the window of opportunity, and (2) the establishment of this window in humans, perhaps choosing cGMP as a biomarker since the attempt to use nitrite/nitrate, measured by chemiluminescence, was frustrating. In summary, there are two opposing concepts: (1) the use of MB as a rescue therapy to treat vasoplegic syndrome and (2) the use of MB as a new adjuvant drug (window 1). There is a possibility that MB does not work (second window) or act too late (third window) when the circulatory shock is metabolically irreversible, with high levels of lactate and uncontrollable metabolic acidosis.

It would be more reasonable to consider MB as an adjuvant medication to be used early (window 1) instead of later (window 3). In the absence of a protocol for the use of MB as adjuvant therapy, persistent vasoplegia and the increased need for vasoconstrictors should be significant signs for the prescription of MB.

In the most critical report in the specialized literature, 36 patients undergoing elective liver transplantation were randomized to receive an intravenous bolus (1.5 mg.Kg^{-1}) before graft reperfusion or saline (placebo). In this study, Koelzow et al. (2003) recorded hemodynamic variables, postoperative liver function tests, and time to hospital discharge. Blood samples were analyzed for arterial lactate concentration, cyclic guanosine-3′,5′-monophosphate, and plasma nitrite/nitrate concentrations. The MB group had higher mean arterial pressure, higher cardiac index, and less need for epinephrine. There was no difference in systemic vascular resistance and central venous pressure. Serum lactate levels were lower than 1 hour after reperfusion in MB patients, suggesting better tissue perfusion. In the presence of MB, there was a reduction in cyclic guanosine-3′,5′-monophosphate, but not in plasma nitrites. Postoperative liver function tests and time to hospital discharge were the same in both groups. These data prove that the MB attenuates the hemodynamic changes of the systemic inflammatory reaction (SIR) in transplantation acting through the inhibition of guanylate cyclase [6].

In Koelzow (2003) cases, MB was used before the perfusion of the transplanted liver, that is, it was used in the prevention of ischemia-reperfusion syndrome. The first case in this condition has only recently been published [6].

The first use of MB as a last resort agent for the adjuvant vasopressor pharmacological treatment in refractory vasoplegic syndrome during liver transplant surgery has been reported. A 61-year-old male patient underwent liver and kidney transplantation due to fulminant hepatorenal failure secondary to autoimmune hepatitis. After reperfusion of the graft, the patient became profoundly hypotensive and required several boluses of calcium chloride, sodium bicarbonate, epinephrine, and norepinephrine. Despite these measures, persistent arterial hypotension (70/50 mmHg) led the anesthesia team to start infusing epinephrine and norepinephrine. The required dose for both infusions was rapidly increased to a maximum of 0.3 µg/kg/min, without any improvement in hemodynamic status. Shortly after that, a vasopressin infusion (4 U/h) was initiated to support blood pressure further, leading only to minimal improvement in hemodynamics. Because the set of hemodynamic data suggests VS, a loading dose of MB was started (2 mg.Kg^{-1} for 30 minutes), followed by a maintenance infusion for 6 hours (0.5 mg/kg/h). Shortly after the start of MB infusion, there was a significant improvement in hemodynamics, allowing the interruption of MB weaning and subsequent infusion of vasopressin and norepinephrine. Blood pressure remained stable at about 100/60 mmHg, with only minimal support for vasoactive amines for the remainder of the process (epinephrine, 0.05 µg/kg/min). The anesthesia group that reported this first case concluded that the number of liver transplant procedures is increasing worldwide and, due to limited clinical experience with MB, many anesthesiologists are unaware of the potential therapeutic effects that this drug can have on the vasoplegic vasculature. This report highlights the benefits of MB administration for the treatment of VS. Therefore, the authors believe that members of the anesthesia team who care for patients undergoing liver transplantation should be aware of its beneficial effects on vasopressor treatment in refractory VS. It is necessary, once again, to emphasize that MB is not a vasopressor drug. In fact, by blocking the cGMP system, it enhances the action of amines in a kind of "cross talk" with the cAMP system linked to the adrenergic system.

Guanylate Cyclase Inhibition in Hepatopulmonary Syndrome

Hepatopulmonary syndrome (HPS) is a triad of liver disease, abnormalities in pulmonary gas exchange leading to arterial hypoxemia, and generalized pulmonary vascular dilation. Both acute and chronic liver diseases have been associated with hepatopulmonary syndrome. Most commonly, the syndrome presents itself in patients with chronic liver disease, resulting in cirrhosis. Portal hypertension seems to be the predominant factor related to this syndrome. The characteristic of vascular changes in pulmonary syndrome is dilated vessels at the levels of precapillary and capillary communications. Direct arteriovenous causes right-to-left communication with a blood flow deviation, incompatibility between ventilation and perfusion, and diffusion limitation. The measurement of PaO$_2$ alone may underestimate the correct degree of oxygenation abnormality due to hyperventilation, which is common in patients with cirrhosis. The alveolar-arterial difference of partial oxygen pressure – D (Aa) O$_2$ – is more accurate, because it includes the determination of PaCO$_2$, which is low, because of hyperventilation [7].

The predominant clinical interest in hepatopulmonary syndrome is based on its relatively high prevalence, which affects 5–29% of patients with terminal liver disease, and a high mortality rate. However this mortality corresponds to 41% for approximately 3 years, but the patients remained clinically stable, despite liver dysfunction, and the failure of numerous medical therapies.

The mechanism underlying this generalized pulmonary vasodilation is unknown. Over the past few years, increasing attention has been focused on NO, a potent local vasodilator that usually contributes to low pulmonary vascular tone. The increase in endogenous NO production has been proposed as an essential determinant of hyperdynamic circulation in cirrhosis. The free radical NO activates soluble guanylate cyclase in vascular smooth muscle, increasing the level of the second messenger cyclic guanosine monophosphate, causing vasorelaxation.

In a case report of a patient with hepatopulmonary syndrome, Schenk et al. (2000) observed an improvement in PaO_2 after the administration of MB. These authors raised the hypothesis that the inhibition of vasodilation was endothelium-dependent. Thus, the inhibition of NO by MB could improve gas exchange and hemodynamic changes in patients with severe hepatopulmonary syndrome. They studied seven patients with advanced cirrhosis and acute hepatopulmonary syndrome with a PaO_2 of 60 mmHg or less. The protocol included the insertion of a pulmonary artery catheter and an arterial catheter before intravenous administration of MB, 3 mg.Kg^{-1} body weight for 15 minutes, controlling serial measurements of gas exchange and hemodynamic variables. The results proved that hypoxemia and hyperdynamic circulation improved in patients with liver cirrhosis and severe hepatopulmonary syndrome. The treatment effect started quickly after intravenous administration of MB and lasted at least 5 hours, e.g., even after 10 hours, oxygenation remained significantly better. The study investigated the effects mainly of MB in patients with severe hepatopulmonary syndrome. PaO_2 normalized in five patients and improved in two patients, with values close to normal. A possible mechanism of MB action may be the inhibition of vasodilation induced by NO, by blocking the soluble guanylate cyclase stimulation, and by its possible action against the superoxide anion generation [8].

Previous studies have already investigated the NO role in cirrhosis. Patients with decompensated cirrhosis have high levels of NO release, including a high concentration of exhaled NO and nitrate levels, compared to patients who have compensated cirrhosis.

MB and NO synthase inhibitors have been shown to block NO-induced vasodilation and thus increase blood pressure and systemic vascular resistance. However, the MB effects on regional blood flow and cardiac contractility were different from those caused by NO synthase inhibitors. The latter caused a decrease in cardiac function and led to adverse effects on organ perfusion. In contrast, MB brought improvements in cardiac function and splanchnic perfusion. Therefore, the option for MB in patients with severe hepatopulmonary syndrome would be more rational.

Liver transplantation is considered a surgical treatment option in patients with hepatopulmonary syndrome since medical treatments, so far, have been disappointing. Such unsatisfactory results have been accompanied by many studies using various pharmaceutical agents such as indomethacin, almitrine, octreotide, and garlic, which have not shown consistently positive effects. Thus, the use of MB should be considered more and may offer a new approach to long-term treatment strategies.

Brief Notes on Transplants from Other Solid Organs

The experience revealed by the specialized literature is small. However, the concepts discussed concerning liver transplantation are extended to other types of solid organ transplants [1].

Kidney Transplant

There are not enough scientific investigations on VS during or after kidney transplantation, to date, to recommend MB routinely to prevent or treat it in this set. Presumably, the preconditions for VS, common in other organ transplants such as cardiac dysfunction, vasopressin deficit, infrared vena cava forceps, or cardiopulmonary bypass, are less frequent or even absent in kidney transplantation. MB should be prescribed carefully after kidney transplantation, as damage to the renal endothelium during early reperfusion is likely to deprive the kidney of the protective vasoactive agents produced by the endothelium of the renal vessels. MB prescribed after renal reperfusion to rescue patients from an unresponsive vascular shock may affect renal function in an unknown way. By inhibiting the GC, MB can deprive the graft of beneficial NO effects, contributing in some way to acute tubular necrosis of the graft [9].

Heart Transplant

NO and MB can interfere with the results of a heart transplant in several different ways. There are many doubts and concerns about the consequences of the NO action or the inhibitions of its effects on acute or chronic graft rejection, coronary vasodilation, oxidative stress, muscle graft contraction, and pulmonary pressure, mainly because there is a shortage of clinical studies [1, 10–12].

Lung Transplant

The lungs are incredibly susceptible to injury, and, despite advances in surgical treatment and immunosuppression, the results of lung transplantation are the worst of any solid organ transplant. High rates of primary graft dysfunction limit the success of lung transplantation due to ischemia-reperfusion injury characterized by robust inflammation, alveolar damage, and vascular permeability [13, 14].

Concluding Remarks

- The NO/cGMP pathway has a significant influence on hemodynamic changes that occur in transplants. Classically, vasoplegic syndrome (VS) is characterized by hypotension and low vascular resistance when guanosine 3'5'-cyclic monophosphate (cGMP) and nitric oxide (NO) increase, contributing to oxidative stress within an inflammatory context.
- The important relationship between graft dysfunction or rejection and ischemia-reperfusion injury is known to be related to the inflammatory response and activation of the NO/cGMP pathway.
- The role of NO in VS in organ transplantation is not known. The number of organ transplant procedures is increasing worldwide. The ischemia and reperfusion syndrome observed during transplant surgery may contribute to a vasoplegic state that often requires vasopressor support to maintain stable hemodynamics.
- The mechanism of hemodynamic instability during organ transplantation is certainly multifactorial, but deregulation of NO production is likely to play an important role. The activation of cGMP production has been associated with hemodynamic instability during liver transplantation.
- The literature describes many clinical cases with the application of methylene blue in the therapeutic approach of shock and vasoplegia, a condition characterized by hypotension and low systemic vascular resistance, refractory to conventional vasopressor therapy.
- It may be that the NO/cGMP pathway has been underestimated due to its important role in the ischemia-reperfusion injury and, consequently, in graft dysfunction. A better understanding of these rejection mechanisms can provide a potential target for future therapies, helping to reduce transplant mortality.
- It is suggested that methylene blue is safe and lifesaving in vasoplegia of resistant amines caused by the reperfusion of organ grafts. Perhaps, it would be wiser to consider MB, not as a delayed rescue treatment, but as an adjuvant drug to be used early (window 1). In the absence of a protocol for the use of MB as an adjuvant therapy, perhaps persistent vasoplegia and the increased need for vasoconstrictors are indicative signs for the use of MB.

References

1. Miranda LE, Mente ED, Fernandes Molina CA, Sumarelli Albuquerque AA, Rubens de Nadai T, Arcencio L, et al. Methylene blue and the NO/cGMP pathway in solid organs transplants. Minerva Anestesiol. 2020;86(4):423–32.
2. Bezinover D, Kadry Z, Uemura T, Sharghi M, Mastro AM, Sosnoski DM, et al. Association between plasma cyclic guanosine monophosphate levels and hemodynamic instability during liver transplantation. Liver Transpl. 2013;19(2):191–8.
3. Miranda LC, Viaro F, Ceneviva R, Evora PR. Endothelium-dependent and -independent hepatic artery vasodilatation is not impaired in a canine model of liver ischemia-reperfusion injury. Braz J Med Biol Res = Rev Bras Pesqui Med Biol. 2007;40(6):857–65.

4. Soares ROS, Losada DM, Jordani MC, Evora P, Castro ESO. Ischemia/reperfusion injury revisited: an overview of the latest pharmacological strategies. Int J Mol Sci. 2019;20(20):5034.
5. Evora PR, Ribeiro PJ, Vicente WV, Reis CL, Rodrigues AJ, Menardi AC, et al. Methylene blue for vasoplegic syndrome treatment in heart surgery: fifteen years of questions, answers, doubts and certainties. Rev Bras Cir Cardiovasc. 2009;24(3):279–88.
6. Koelzow H, Gedney JA, Baumann J, Snook NJ, Bellamy MC. The effect of methylene blue on the hemodynamic changes during ischemia reperfusion injury in orthotopic liver transplantation. Anesth Analg. 2002;94(4):824–9, table of contents.
7. Thevenot T, Pastor CM, Cervoni JP, Jacquelinet C, Nguyen-Khac E, Richou C, et al. [Hepatopulmonary syndrome]. Gastroenterol Clin Biol. 2009;33(6–7):565–79.
8. Schenk P, Madl C, Rezaie-Majd S, Lehr S, Muller C. Methylene blue improves the hepatopulmonary syndrome. Ann Intern Med. 2000;133(9):701–6.
9. Rhoden EL, Rhoden CR, Lucas ML, Pereira-Lima L, Zettler C, Bello-Klein A. The role of nitric oxide pathway in the renal ischemia-reperfusion injury in rats. Transpl Immunol. 2002;10(4):277–84.
10. Pieper GM, Roza AM. The complex role of iNOS in acutely rejecting cardiac transplants. Free Radic Biol Med. 2008;44(8):1536–52.
11. Kofidis T, Struber M, Wilhelmi M, Anssar M, Simon A, Harringer W, et al. Reversal of severe vasoplegia with single-dose methylene blue after heart transplantation. J Thorac Cardiovasc Surg. 2001;122(4):823–4.
12. Grubb KJ, Kennedy JL, Bergin JD, Groves DS, Kern JA. The role of methylene blue in serotonin syndrome following cardiac transplantation: a case report and review of the literature. J Thorac Cardiovasc Surg. 2012;144(5):e113–6.
13. Laubach VE, Sharma AK. Mechanisms of lung ischemia-reperfusion injury. Curr Opin Organ Transplant. 2016;21(3):246–52.
14. Abreu Mda M, Pazetti R, Almeida FM, Correia AT, Parra ER, Silva LP, et al. Methylene blue attenuates ischemia--reperfusion injury in lung transplantation. J Surg Res. 2014;192(2):635–41.

Chapter 17
Acid-Base Balance

Alkalosis occurs due to a reduction in partial pressure of carbon dioxide (PCO_2) in situations that cause respiratory hyperventilation or an increase in the number of bases observed in conditions such as persistent vomiting, gastric aspiration, use of diuretics, adrenal hyperactivity, as well as administration of alkalis for the treatment of acidosis during cardiopulmonary bypass, pulmonary hypertension, cardiac arrest, and others.

The endothelium can regulate vascular tone under the influence of intra- or extracellular pH. Thus, alkalosis can induce contraction or relaxation, depending on the type of vessel and the species. How acid-base shifts are caused (change in PCO_2 or addition of acid and base) is also essential to the kind of vascular response produced. In addition to its direct effect on vascular tone, alkalosis can also alter vascular responsiveness to vasoconstricting and vasodilating agents.

The mechanisms by which alkalosis influences vascular tone or its response to specific agonists are not yet fully understood. However, there is some evidence that suggest the participation of nitric oxide (NO), prostacyclin (PGI2), potassium channels, and calcium flow [1].

Cellular metabolism produces acids that are continuously released into intra- and extracellular fluids and tend to modify the concentration of hydrogen ions (H^+). The maintenance of the concentration of H^+ ions within the optimum range for cellular metabolism depends on the elimination of carbonic acid by the lungs, H^+ ions by the kidneys, and the action of the intra- and extracellular buffer systems. How the body regulates the concentration of H^+ ions is of fundamental importance for understanding and assessing changes in the balance between acids and bases within cells in the surrounding liquid medium (interstitial fluid) and in the blood (intravascular fluid).

Hydrogen potency (pH) is the term used to measure the concentration of free H^+ ions in solution. Blood pH is maintained under standard conditions within the range of 7.35–7.45. This variation is essential for the regular activity of the organism. The maintenance of the ideal amount of these H^+ ions in the intra- and extracellular liquids depends on a delicate chemical balance between the acids and bases in the body called the acid-base balance.

© The Author(s), under exclusive license to Springer Nature
Switzerland AG 2021
P. R. Barbosa Evora et al., *Vasoplegic Endothelial Dysfunction*,
https://doi.org/10.1007/978-3-030-74096-2_17

Acid-basic homeostasis occurs due to the daily production of organic acids by the metabolism; consequently, an efficient buffering system is necessary so that there is no loss of this balance; in this sense, the main organs related to the buffer system are the lungs and kidneys. When this balance is broken, changes called acidemia (acidosis) and alkalemia (alkalosis) occur. These terms indicate changes in the concentration of H^+ ions in the blood. Acidemia means pH below 7.35, and alkalemia means pH above 7.45.

In addition to the critical role of the lungs and kidneys in maintaining homeostasis, the blood has efficient defense mechanisms against sudden or significant changes in pH, resisting changes in its normality through pairs of substances that are capable of reacting with both acids and bases. These physiological actions are called "buffer" systems, and, as defense mechanisms, they also exist in the intracellular and interstitial fluid.

Tampons are substances that limit the pH variations of blood and other organic liquids when combined with the acids or bases present in these liquids. The plugs are composed of substances that act in pairs constituting a protective system. The buffer system consists of a weak acid and its salt, formed with a strong base. The weak acid and salt in the buffer system, under normal conditions, exist in a constant relationship, which the body tends to preserve. The primary body buffers are sodium bicarbonate, acidic and essential proteins, hemoglobin, and phosphate.

All body fluids have buffer systems to prevent significant pH changes. When an acid accumulates in the body, it is neutralized in the blood, in the interstitial fluid and inside the cells, and in approximately equal parts, the intracellular process being slower because it takes about 2 hours to compensate for a change.

The balance of intracellular pH occurs differently from blood pH since cell activity permanently generates acidic by-products due to cell metabolism. Thus, the pH of the intracellular liquid is lower than the pH of the plasma, reaching values close to 6.9 in the cells, about 7.3 in the renal tubular cells, and varying between 6.9 and 7.3 in the other cells. In general, tissue cells with higher metabolic activity have a slightly acidic pH, compared to the blood pH. Respiratory mechanisms are of crucial importance in regulating the pH of body fluids in the face of sudden changes in the balance between acids and bases. Blood pH can modify alveolar ventilation through the respiratory center to maintain the body's homeostasis. The respiratory center acts as a "sensor" of the blood pH, that is, when the concentration of H^+ in the blood is high (low pH), the respiratory center increases the respiratory rate by eliminating an enormous amount of carbon dioxide (CO_2) and raising the pH to normal levels. Conversely, when the H^+ concentration is low (high pH), the respiratory center decreases the respiratory rate, retaining CO_2 and reducing the pH to normal levels.

The role of the kidneys in regulating the concentration of H^+ ions occurs by increasing or decreasing the level of bicarbonate ions in body fluids. The amount of bicarbonate ions is regulated by the reactions that take place in the renal tubules. These reactions involve CO_2, water, and an enzyme called carbonic anhydrase.

The body does not tolerate pronounced changes in pH well. Values below 6.8 or above 7.8 are challenging to reverse. Depending on the source, disturbances in the acid-base balance (acidosis or alkalosis) can be of a metabolic or respiratory nature.

Cellular metabolism promotes the accumulation of acids that reduce the pH of the blood, characterizing a metabolic (non-respiratory) acidosis. When the body accumulates CO_2 due to inadequate ventilation, the pH is reduced, and acidosis is of respiratory origin. If the body accumulates excess bases, for example, bicarbonate, the pH rises, characterizing that alkalosis is of metabolic origin. However, if the body eliminates excess CO_2, the pH increases, characterizing a situation of respiratory alkalosis.

The laboratory value found in acidosis is pH below 7.35, which characterizes acidosis. PCO_2 above 45 mmHg means respiratory disturbance or changes in bicarbonate. In addition, it is known that changes in extracellular pH (pH0) promote changes in vascular tone, which affects circulation and blood pressure control. Gaskell (1880) was probably the first to show that pH is essential for vascular tone when he demonstrated, in a frog mesenteric artery, that a reduction in pH using lactic acid led to an increase in vascular diameter, while an increase at pH by sodium hydroxide promoted a decrease in vascular diameter [2, 3].

When pH0 is in the range of 7.4, the intracellular pH (pHi) in the vascular smooth muscle cell is around 7.1. Due to the flow of ions through the cell membrane, changes in pH0 reflect changes in pHi in the same direction, but with different speed, duration, and intensity. For example, in myocytes, the displacement of pH0 changes pHi by 30% in relation to pH0 within 10–40 minutes. However, in the mesenteric artery, changes in pHi are around 70% in relation to pH0 and occur within just 2 minutes.

The measurement of pH0 is relatively simple, both in vivo (blood gas analysis) and in vitro (electrode connected to pH-meter). However, the pHi measure is more complicated and started to be performed in the 1980s using magnetic resonance techniques and fluorescence indicator probes (2'7'-bis-carboxyethyl-5 (6)-carboxy-fluorescein (BCECF) and 5-(and-6)-carboxy SNARF®-1, acetoxymethyl ester, acetate) [4]. The magnetic resonance imaging method can be used for vascular tissue but due to factors, such as the need for a minimum tissue mass of 500 mg, high cost, and low-resolution time, has not been the method of choice for most researchers. Fluorescence indicators have been widely used to measure intracellular pH, as they are more sensitive and can be used even in a single cell.

The reduction of perivascular pH in acidemia decreases the responsiveness to vasoconstrictors and results in difficulty in maintaining systemic blood pressure. Perivascular pH can affect many cellular processes, but the precise mechanism of this vascular hyporesponsiveness remains unknown. Changes in pH (7.4–7.0) have shown substantial inhibition of vascular smooth muscle contractility, which has been associated with increased hyperpolarization and storage of Ca^{+2} in intracellular organelles.

The mechanisms by which pH influences vascular tone or its response to specific agonists may involve NO, prostacyclin (PGI-2), potassium, and calcium channels. For example, in a rat aorta, reductions in intracellular pH can affect the intracellular concentration of Ca^{+2}, by mechanisms that involve an influx of Ca^{+2} into the sarcoplasmic reticulum. Changes in pH can also act directly on contractile myofilaments and alter the receptors on the cell membrane.

Influence of Alkalinization on Vascular Reactivity

Studies carried out in a rat mesenteric artery showed that intracellular alkalinization by trimethylamine promoted vasoconstriction. The same effect was observed for extracellular alkalinization with sodium hydroxide (NaOH). Likewise, intracellular alkalinization with ammonium chloride (NH_4Cl) also induced vasoconstriction in a pig's coronary artery and dog's intrapulmonary artery. In a rat cerebral artery, intracellular alkalinization by NH_4Cl or trimethylamine did not promote any change in vascular tone. The same was observed for the dog pulmonary artery and rabbits, as well as in a rabbit aorta, in which no changes in vascular tone were observed due to changes in pHi [1].

When the Vessel Studied Was the Rat Aorta, Intracellular Alkalinization Promoted the Same Sustained Contraction

Using alkalosis in a pig's pulmonary artery as a stimulus, vasodilation was also observed, whose mechanism involves NO, PGI2, and K^+ channel activated by Ca^{+2}. However, when the vessel under study was the pulmonary vein, only NO was involved in alkalinization-induced vasodilation (PCO_2 reduction).

The alkalinization induced by sodium bicarbonate in a rabbit basilar artery promoted vasoconstriction. The same effect was observed for alkalinization with NaOH in the rabbit basilar artery and rat cerebral artery by the reduction in arterial diameter [1].

Gordon et al. (2003) showed, in the porcine pulmonary artery, that alkalinization by reducing PCO_2 in a precontracted vessel with U46619 (thromboxane analog) promoted NO-dependent vasodilation since the addition of N^G-monomethyl-L-arginine (L-NMMA) inhibited this. However, the same alkalinizing stimulus in the endothelium of the aorta did not alter the expression of the nitric oxide synthase (NOS) enzyme or the production of guanosine 3′5′-cyclic monophosphate (cGMP) [2].

Studies carried out in a human pulmonary artery endothelial cell showed that when placed in an alkaline medium (pH 8.0), they present an increase in the expression of the enzyme NOS and exchanger Na^+/Ca^{+2}. The authors also suggest that there may be an interaction between the Na^+/Ca^{+2} exchanger and NOS in the control of pulmonary circulation.

The direct, or even indirect, effect of pH on vascular tone due to the influence on the action of agonists is still poorly understood. Different vascular beds in different species have appropriate responses to both acidification and alkalinization. However, it is possible to say that at least one of the following mechanisms is involved in the vascular effects triggered by changes in pH: NO, PGI2, Ca^{+2} channels, and K^+ channels.

Influence of Chronic Metabolic Acidosis and Vascular Reactivity

Chronic ammonium chloride (NH_4Cl)-induced metabolic acidosis causes harmful effects on cardiac function by reducing cardiac output and stroke volume, without altering the heart rate. In the vascular reactivity of rat carotids, it enhanced the relaxation induced by calcium ionophore in a manner dependent on NO, and no changes were observed for the other tested agonists. It also reduced plasma nitrite and nitrate levels. In the assessment of respiratory parameters, it caused increased ventilation and tidal volume, without causing changes in respiratory rate. However, there were no changes in urea and creatinine and kidney morphology.

Disorders in the acid-base balance are problems commonly found in clinical medicine, and decisions regarding its treatment are of great importance in patients with lung problems, in which these disorders can be especially critical. Likewise, in the face of acid-base disorders, the cardiopulmonary function may be significantly impaired, even in patients without intrinsic heart or lung disease. Therefore, it is essential to understand the pathophysiological consequences of these disorders on the cardiovascular and pulmonary systems.

Since Gaskell (1880) studied the tonicity of blood vessels in acidic solution, it was recognized that blood pH, among other factors such as hypoxia and PCO_2, is an important determinant of vascular tone [3].

Moreover, the vasodilator effect of acidosis has been investigated in different types of vascular beds. The literature shows that acidosis causes changes in vascular responsiveness to different agonists. However, these results are obtained in models of acidosis in vitro. In these cases, most studies indicate decreased contraction or enhanced relaxation mediated by NO and potassium channels.

Studies by Celotto et al. (2016) in rabbits, using the acute and chronic acidosis model, observed that only acute acidosis promoted an increase in the acetylcholine (ACh) hypotensive effect in vivo [4]. However, when the arteries (aorta and carotid) of acidotic animals were placed in an organ bath, their changes in reactivity were observed for ACh and phenylephrine (Phe), corroborating with the results found by Magalhães et al. (2016), who also found no changes in reactivity to ACh in the renal artery of acidotic rats. In this study, it was observed that only relaxation induced by calcium ionophore (A23187) was enhanced by acidosis [5]. Such effect was observed in the presence of endothelium and blocked by N^G-Nitro-L-Arginine Methyl Ester (L-NAME), suggesting the NO participation. The mechanism by which ionophore calcium promotes relaxation involves increasing the influx of calcium into the endothelial cell, activating the calcium-calmodulin pathway, and inducing the production of NO that diffuses into the muscle promoting relaxation. The literature shows that increasing the concentration of extracellular H^+ can alter the functioning of pumps and exchangers present in the cell membrane, such as Na^+/K^+-ATPase, Na^+/Ca^{2+} exchanger (NCX), Ca^{2+} channel type L (LCC), Na^+/H^+ exchanger (NHE), Ca^{2+} release channel from the sarcoplasmic reticulum (SR) (ryanodine receptor, RyR), and SR Ca^+-ATPase (SERCA). We could consider that acidosis can alter the functioning of the NHE exchange, which alters the sodium concentration, leading to an inversion of the NCX and an increase in intracellular Ca^{2+} in the endothelium. This accumulation of Ca^{2+} induced by acidosis could, in addition to Ca^{2+} mobilized by calcium ionophore, increase NOS activity and vascular NO production. The absence of changes for ACh and the other vasoconstrictors suggests that there is no endothelial dysfunction, nor changes in the expression and function of AT-1, α-adrenergic, and ET-A receptors. Biais et al. (2012) showed that only the signaling linked to beta-adrenergic receptors is altered, an effect that was not observed for signaling involving alpha-adrenergic receptors [6]. Although an increase in arterial NO induced by calcium ionophore can be observed, we did not observe an increase in plasma NO, as would be expected for acidosis.

On the contrary, a decrease in plasma nitrite and nitrate was observed, which did not impair vascular relaxation. Celotto et al. (2009) noted in an acidosis model in rabbits that only acute acidosis promoted an increase in plasma NO, an effect not observed in the chronic model. Some factors could justify the decrease in NO in acidosis: One is that, initially, the acid medium allows more excellent NO stability and, therefore, more time of action. Its products also tend to be converted back to NO that could imply a decrease in NO production since it remains available for a longer time, with less NO being sufficient to perform its role. Another factor is that acidosis and oxidative stress intensify each other. Acidosis can also lead to oxidative stress by lowering the intracellular levels of one of the most critical antioxidants, glutathione, a decrease achieved through multiple pH-related mechanisms. Acidosis can also reduce the activity of antioxidant enzymes. Thus, higher NO consumption by reactive species could be occurring [7].

Acute Acidosis Compared to Chronic Acidosis

Metabolic acidosis has profound effects on vascular tone. A study of our authorship investigated the in vivo effects of acute metabolic acidosis (AMA) and chronic metabolic acidosis (CMA) on hemodynamic parameters and endothelial function.

CMA was induced by ad libitum intake of 1% NH_4Cl for 7 days, and AMA was induced by a 3-hour infusion of 6 M NH_4Cl (1 mL/kg, diluted 1:10). The dose-response curves of phenylephrine (Phe) and acetylcholine (ACh) were performed by venous infusion with simultaneous monitoring of venous and arterial blood pressure. Plasma nitrite/nitrate (NOx) was measured by chemiluminescence.

The CMA group had a blood pH of 7.15 ± 0.03, associated with a reduction in bicarbonate (13.8 ± 0.98 mmol/L) and no change in the partial arterial carbon dioxide ($PaCO_2$) pressure. The AMA group had a pH of 7.20 ± 0.01, associated with reductions in bicarbonate (10.8 ± 0.54 mmol/L) and $PaCO_2$ (47.8 ± 2.54 to 23.2 ± 0.74 mmHg) and accompanied by hyperventilation. The infusion of Phe or ACh did not affect the blood or venous pressure in the CMA group. However, the ACh infusion decreased the blood pressure (ΔBP: −28.0 ± 2.35 mm Hg (AMA) to −4.5 ± 2.89 mmHg (control)) in the AMA group. Plasma NOx was normal after

CMA but increased after AMA (25.3 ± 0.88 to 31.3 ± 0.54 µM). These results indicate that AMA, but not CMA, potentiates ACh-induced blood pressure decrease and leads to an increase in plasma NOx, reinforcing the effect of pH imbalance on the control of vascular tone and blood pressure [4].

Acidosis and Inflammation

Abnormalities in the systemic acid-base balance can induce significant changes in the immune response and can play a vital role in the development or maintenance of immune dysfunction. Different forms of acidosis (metabolic and respiratory) and even different types of metabolic acidosis (hyperchloremic and lactic) can produce different effects on immune function. However, whether alkalinization has an impact on controlling inflammation is still a matter of speculation.

Most of the time, metabolic acidosis is present in the acute systemic inflammatory response, in which the control of acid-base balance is part of the treatment protocol. Thus, the assessment of the metabolic acidosis role is mandatory. One of the main concerns about this article is the difficulty of establishing "Which came first, the chicken or the egg?"

In many cases, acute acidosis is secondary to, for example, circulatory shock, and one can ask whether, under these conditions, the circulatory shock causes the inflammatory response or shock-related acidosis. The same reasoning can be followed in patients who develop respiratory acidosis due to acute respiratory distress syndrome (ARDS) or chronic obstructive pulmonary disorder COPD, as lung disease alone induces an inflammatory response.

Perhaps the most unambiguous data that provide evidence of an impaired immune response appear in clinical studies of organic acidosis and ketoacidosis. In general, clinical acidemias are accompanied by immunodeficiency, including a reduction in the number of white blood cells, gamma globulins, mitogenic responses, decreased inflammatory response, and delayed phagocytosis. In many cases, immunodeficiency is reversed in the correction of acidosis. However, despite the valuable research carried out to date, there is a lack of appreciation of the extracellular effects of acid-base in a wide range of other immunological activities. Therefore, situations in which acidosis remains constant, such as chronic renal failure, would be more appropriate for evaluating treatment to contain the spread of the inflammatory process.

It should be emphasized that metabolic acidosis is common in critically ill patients and its presence can have a detrimental effect on the clinical outcome. The administration of the base, a common therapeutic maneuver, does not significantly improve the clinical result, even when the acidosis is improved.

Concluding Remarks

- Metabolic acidosis is one of the most common abnormalities in patients suffering from serious illnesses, and there is growing evidence to suggest that acidosis itself has profound effects on the host, especially on immune function.
- Recent evidence suggests that different forms of acidosis (metabolic and respiratory) and even different types of metabolic acidosis (hyperchloremic and lactic) can produce different effects on immune function.
- The publications that link acidosis with the inflammatory response are limited, and a major criticism of experimental studies is strong acidification (pH 6.5–7.0), which most clearly shows the role of inflammation, and these levels of acidosis are rarely observed in the clinical setting.
- Anion gap, bicarbonate, and lactate are possible biomarkers of the response to inflammation.
- Perhaps the most unambiguous data that provide evidence of impaired immune response emerges from clinical studies of organic acidosis and ketoacidosis. In general, clinical acidemias are accompanied by immunodeficiency, including a reduction in the number of white cells, gamma globulins and mitogenic responses, and a decrease in the inflammatory response.
- Currently, considering the inflammatory response, to consider which are the best strategies for the treatment of metabolic acidosis is an exercise of speculation and hypothesis.
- Administration of selective NHE1 inhibitors minimizes the degree of cell damage and improves survival.
- The correction of metabolic acidosis as an isolated marker needs to be abandoned and should be considered an essential part of the systemic inflammatory response.

References

1. Celotto AC, Capellini VK, Baldo CF, Dalio MB, Rodrigues AJ, Evora PR. Effects of acid-base imbalance on vascular reactivity. Braz J Med Biol Res = Rev Bras Pesqui Med Biol. 2008;41(6):439–45.
2. Gordon JB, VanderHeyden MA, Halla TR, Cortez EP, Hernandez G, Haworth ST, et al. What leads to different mediators of alkalosis-induced vasodilation in isolated and in situ pulmonary vessels? Am J Physiol Lung Cell Mol Physiol. 2003;284(5):L799–807.
3. Gaskell WH. On the tonicity of the heart and blood vessels. J Physiol. 1880;3(1):48–92 16.
4. Celotto AC, Ferreira LG, Capellini VK, Albuquerque AA, Rodrigues AJ, Evora PR. Acute but not chronic metabolic acidosis potentiates the acetylcholine-induced reduction in blood pressure: an endothelium-dependent effect. Braz J Med Biol Res = Rev Bras Pesqui Med Biol. 2016;49(2):e5007.
5. Magalhaes PA, de Brito TS, Freire RS, da Silva MT, dos Santos AA, Vale ML, et al. Metabolic acidosis aggravates experimental acute kidney injury. Life Sci. 2016;146:58–65.

6. Biais M, Jouffroy R, Carillion A, Feldman S, Jobart-Malfait A, Riou B, et al. Interaction of metabolic and respiratory acidosis with alpha and beta-adrenoceptor stimulation in rat myocardium. Anesthesiology. 2012;117(6):1212–22.
7. Celotto AC, Capellini VK, Baldo CF, Restini CB, Evora PR. Extracellular acidosis promote endothelium-independent and nitric oxide-dependent vasodilation. FASEB J. 2009;23(S1):952.13.

Chapter 18
The Therapeutic Use of Inhaled Nitric Oxide

Mechanisms of Action

Hypertension in the pulmonary vascular circulation may be due to a postcapillary obstruction or an increase in flow that leads to secondary alterations such as muscle layer proliferation, fibrosis, and light obliteration. Also, nitric oxide (NO) inhalation can be valuable in the management, reducing the work imposed on the right ventricle and improving oxygenation [1].

Due to the rapid inactivation caused by hemoglobin and its short half-life, inhaled NO should activate selective pulmonary vasodilation when there is vasoconstriction, secondary to endothelial dysfunction, or because of an abundant vasoconstrictor influence.

NO should allow better oxygenation when administered in the presence of a balanced infusion and ventilation. Therefore, there are advantages over endogenously administered vasodilators that cause hypotension and increase intrapulmonary shunt [1].

The effectiveness of inhaled NO as a pulmonary vasodilator in patients where endothelial damage is associated with the disease state raises the question of whether the endogenously released NO deficiency is responsible for the increase in pulmonary vascular tone. NO would be released continuously below baseline conditions, and inhibition of these basal release conditions could lead to increased vascular resistance. Perfusion of human lungs alone with methylene blue (MB), an inhibitor of NO-mediated vasorelaxation, leads to an increase in pulmonary vascular resistance. Thus, endothelial damage, with a reduction of intravenous NO, should be considered when pulmonary vasoconstriction is a consequence of the disease (e.g., respiratory distress syndrome in adults – ARDS) or a transient side effect of the treatment (e.g., cardiopulmonary bypass).

Inhaled NO, unlike intravenous NO, has a limited action on veins and arteries of small resistance, and it is impossible to dilate large-capacity vessels. In lungs

P. R. Barbosa Evora et al., *Vasoplegic Endothelial Dysfunction*, https://doi.org/10.1007/978-3-030-74096-2_18

perfused with inhaled NO, arterial vessels are primarily affected, but during extreme venous vasoconstriction, it can also act at the postcapillary level. In adults with acute lung disease, NO has a predominantly vasodilating effect on pulmonary venous vascularization. This increase in responsiveness appears in pediatric patients with pulmonary venous hypertension, in which NO must result in vasodilation with a combination of pre- and postcapillary vessels [1].

The occurrence of right ventricular failure secondary to pulmonary arterial hypertension is the main postoperative complication of cardiac surgery in children and adults. The selective pulmonary vasodilation produced by inhaled NO is a therapeutic option that, in certain situations, can be fundamental in the administration of this condition. NO binds to hemoglobin, resulting in its immediate inactivation, resulting in the maintenance of systemic and coronary blood pressures (Fig. 18.1).

Technical and Ethical Aspects

NO is toxic when inhaled at high levels. It produces methemoglobinemia and lung damage primarily by oxidation to nitrogen dioxide (NO_2). International experiences have shown significant pulmonary vasodilation in patients breathing low concentrations of 5–40 ppm, levels that do not appear to be toxic. The use of 80 ppm for

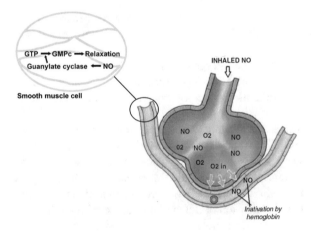

Fig. 18.1 Schematic representation of the mechanism and site of action of inhaled nitric oxide (NO). Inhaled NO action, different from the NO intravenous action, is limited to veins and arteries of small resistance and is unable to dilate large capacitance vessels. In lungs inhaled NO acts primarily on the arterial vessels but can, during extreme venous vasoconstriction, also act in the postcapillary bed. The selective pulmonary vasodilation produced by inhaled NO is a therapeutic option. NO binds to hemoglobin, resulting in its systemic inactivation and resulting in maintenance of coronary and systemic blood pressures. In acute lung injuries, inhaled NO is preferably released in areas where ventilation is high. Blood vessels are affected by hypoxic vasoconstriction in the vicinity of poorly ventilated alveoli. Inhaled NO, under these conditions, redirects pulmonary blood flow to dilated vessels near well-ventilated alveoli, decreases intrapulmonary shunt, and improves oxygenation

3 hours kept the levels of methemoglobin below 3%. Isolated cases, referred to in the literature, showed that the use of NO by inhalation up to 53 days was not associated with high levels of methemoglobin. NO cannot be used intravenously because it is rapidly inactivated by hemoglobin. This aspect makes the inhalation route quite safe for the patient since possible excesses of the absorbed gas are "sequestered" by hemoglobin. However, there are population subgroups with changes in the ability to reduce intra-erythrocyte methemoglobin. The possibility that these groups are more vulnerable to methemoglobinemia, when exposed to NO, warns of the risks of extrapolating data obtained in Europe or the USA to potentially different populations [1].

Regarding the clinical use of NO, a mandatory concern is related to the safety of medical and paramedical personnel involved in patient care due to the toxic NO_2 effects. The US Occupational Safety and Health Administration (OSHA) establishes that inhalation above 25 ppm of NO is permissible within a work environment over 8 hours a day with periodic increases of up to 100 ppm. Some safety measures have already been established: (1) Use aluminum cylinders in the proportion 400–500 ppm of NO supplemented with N2, which reduces the chance of toxic effects, even in the case of total gas leakage due to valve defects; (2) use soda lime on the inspiratory line of the respirator to neutralize NO_2; (3) administer low NO concentrations (<80 ppm); (4) do not use compressed (humid) air from the hospital network in the predilution because the reaction of NO_2 with water forms nitric acid, which is extremely corrosive; (5) add the NO in the circuit previous to the blender of the ventilator (the introduction in the inspiratory branch brings uncertainties and risks to the mixture); (6) do not manufacture your NO for clinical use [1].

Like any new therapeutic modality, the clinical use of NO by inhalation must be approved by the medical ethics committees. Preliminary results are promising, but possible side effects in the short and long term require evaluation by monitoring patients undergoing this treatment. For example, it is known that NO is used as an index of ambient air pollution, and its effects on carcinogenesis are not known. It is not known whether the beneficial effects in the acute phase are permanent or leave sequelae. From a biochemical point of view, it is known that NO can react with superoxide radicals forming the peroxynitrite anion. The decomposition of this anion leads to the formation of a powerful oxidizer with characteristics of the hydroxyl radical, which is toxic. Anyway, the clinical application is justified by the high mortality of the diseases involved. What is not warranted is the indiscriminate use before its real efficiency and safety are established.

The minimum required for its clinical use includes: (1) aluminum cylinders with 400–500 ppm/N2; (2) connection valves that guarantee the integrity of the respirator; (3) availability of methemoglobin dosage; (4) chemiluminescence device for dosing NO and NO_2 at the bedside; (5) special circuit for NO since it is corrosive. The experimental phase requires hemodynamic monitoring at the bedside and trained personnel for the project.

In addition to methemoglobinemia, the possible toxic NO_2 effects and peroxynitrite, and a possible association with carcinogenesis, three other adverse effects must be considered: a possible worsening of left ventricular dysfunction, a rebound of pulmonary hypertension when suspending NO inhalation, and the possibility of coagulopathy due to NO antiplatelet effects.

Critical Analysis

A free analysis based on information, extracted up to 1996, from the two most essential reference banks (Current Contents and Medline) for researching the medical literature, in addition to data from specialized congresses, allows to enumerate some of the main data regarding the use of inhaled NO: (a) Inhaled NO is currently recognized as a valuable pharmacological resource in neonatal and pediatric intensive care and for cardiopulmonary surgery; (b) other applications in adults, such as chronic obstructive pulmonary disease and adult acute respiratory distress syndrome, require careful observation; (c) inhaled NO therapy is relatively inexpensive, but it should be used in all patients, based on the paradigms of its efficiency and potential toxicity; (d) the recent discoveries of its anti-inflammatory and extrapulmonary effects open new horizons for future applications [1].

In addition to this general postulation, a critical analysis, although not intending to address all aspects of the use of inhaled NO in cardiac surgery, should include some questions and possible answers. These questions were based on selected papers [2–7]:

1. *Are there any advantages of using inhaled NO over hyperventilation to control pulmonary hypertension after surgical correction of congenital heart disease?*

   At first, yes. Inhaled NO and hyperventilation are both effective in reducing pulmonary artery pressure (PAP) and pulmonary vascular resistance (PVR). However, the selective action of inhaled NO in the pulmonary circulation offers advantages over hyperventilation because the drop in cardiac output and the increase in systemic vascular resistance (SVR) are undesirable in this period [2]. It should be noted that NO in oxygen appears to be a more potent pulmonary vasodilator than oxygen alone [3].

2. *Can inhaled NO be efficient to increase survival in surgeries for congenital or acquired heart disease with pulmonary hypertension?*

   Although inhaled NO can reduce pulmonary hypertension, it appears that this action is not associated with more prolonged survival. A randomized study is necessary to determine the exact role of inhaled NO in the survival of patients with residual pulmonary hypertension after surgical treatment [4].

3. *Are there subgroups of congenital heart diseases that can obtain better benefits from the use of inhaled NO?*

   The answer is no. Studies show that inhaled NO causes minimal benefit over PAP or cardiac output (CO) in children after correction of the atrioventricular canal [5].

4. *Is it possible to predict the need for the use of inhaled NO in the postoperative period of congenital and acquired heart diseases?*

Some factors have already been associated as predictive of the use of inhaled NO: age <1 year, Down syndrome, preoperative pulmonary hypertension, and increased pulmonary vascular resistance. Seventy-three percent of patients who used inhaled NO were identified, using a multivariate model based on these factors, in a service that allows the unrestricted use of inhaled NO, and 50% of children operated for congenital heart disease have used it [6].

5. *Can inhaled NO be associated with the use of prostacyclins?*

There are some controversies. The combination of both vasodilators was not more potent than the isolated use of iloprost or inhaled NO, both for pharmacological tests and for the control of pulmonary hypertension. Beraprost seems to be a therapeutic alternative to the use of inhaled NO and tolazoline, to study the pulmonary vasodilator response. The combined use of both could be a therapeutic alternative, without significant complications in the treatment of pulmonary hypertension in children [7, 8].

6. *Is there a therapeutic resource against pulmonary hypertension "rebound" after the suspension of inhaled NO?*

Dipyridamole could mitigate rebound pulmonary hypertension after discontinuing the use of inhaled NO in the postoperative period of congenital heart disease. Dipyridamole can support cGMP elevations induced by inhaled NO. Also, phosphodiesterase activity could contribute to acute pulmonary hypertension after suspending inhaled NO [9].

7. *Considering the toxic potential of inhaled NO, are there follow-up studies in the medium and long term of patients submitted to its therapeutic use?*

These studies are still infrequent in the literature. A Japanese study, reporting follow-up of 65 children over 2.0–4.3 years (average 3.1 years), states that all children no longer needed to use oxygen. Also, possible adverse effects, including the occurrence of malignant tumors or chronic inflammation of the respiratory tract, have not been observed [10].

8. *In addition to the reduction in pulmonary vascular resistance, are there any other effects of inhaled NO that can be evaluated from a therapeutic point of view?*

Other actions of inhaled NO should increase interest in its therapeutic potential: Inhaled NO attenuates the proliferation of vascular smooth muscle, inhibits platelet aggregation, and promotes cytoprotection for donor organs, improving the harmful aspects of ischemia-reperfusion damage. Also, it should promote angiogenesis in immature lungs and improve the ability to carry oxygen by hemoglobin in sickle cell anemia [11].

9. *Would it be possible or logical to use NO donor drugs through the inhalation route as an option to inhaled NO?*

At least one published study indicates that nitroglycerin nebulization is effective, inexpensive, and safe to control pulmonary hypertension associated with congenital heart diseases in services that do not have the resources for extracorporeal oxygenation and inhaled NO [12]. In the ICU of the Hospital do Coração of Ribeirão Preto and the Neonatal ICU of the Hospital das Clínicas in Ribeirão Preto, sodium nitroprusside by inhalation has already been used in isolated and desperate cases. Completely randomly, some neonates transiently presented vasodilation and became stained. In some cases, no effect was observed. Sodium nitroprusside was used in an adult patient with severe right ventricular dysfunction secondary to pulmonary hypertension associated with interatrial communication and pulmonary thromboembolism. In the postoperative period of pulmonary thromboendarterectomy, 7 years after the atrial septal defect (ASD) correction, pulmonary hypertension levels reached 180 mmHg. Intravenous sodium nitroprusside reduced pulmonary arterial pressure but was associated with severe systemic arterial hypotension. When the inhalation route was attempted, the blood pressure gave way, but the same happened with the systemic pressure, although in a smaller magnitude than the venous route. It was not possible to conclude whether systemic arterial hypotension was associated with cardiac function or if there was systemic absorption of nitroprusside used by inhalation.

Given the revised aspects, where many controversies are evident, what would be the possible conclusions? One thing is right. Although inhaled NO is proven to be a selective pulmonary vasodilator and, without a doubt, has been saving lives, its use has not become unanimous over more than 10 years, indeed, due to its potential toxicity and to its variability of response (observed, even, in the scope of general neonatology). These events do not encourage the performance of extensive trials, which could clarify many of the controversies mentioned above.

In the early 1990s, one of the authors (PRBE) visited prestigious American clinics (Mayo Clinic, Cleveland Clinic, Johns Hopkins, and Harvard), where clinical experiments with inhaled NO began. A summary of the observations and interviews at these clinics highlighted: (a) the effectiveness of treatment in isolated cases; (b) the variability of the therapeutic response regardless of age, heart, or respiratory disease; (c) better therapeutic response, albeit transitory, in cases of more severe and chronic pulmonary hypertension; (d) the belief that inhaled NO would be a potential therapeutic weapon in transient hypertension, thus neonatology and cardiopulmonary transplants could be benefited; and (e) everyone was apprehensive about the potential NO toxicity, not only for patients but also for professionals who used it. It seems that in more than a decade, these observations are still current and pertinent. Only a consensus appears to be established, namely, the use of smaller doses (10–20 ppm) than those initially used.

Its use has not become unanimous, with the groups that most benefit being those in whom pulmonary hypertension is transient. It is essential to note the relatively small number of reports, many associated with isolated cases, and a considerable prevalence of observation in humans without a substantial experimental basis. This may be due, in part, to the difficulty of obtaining innovative models of pulmonary hypertension, but certainly to the unknown as to the long-term toxic effects of inhaled NO and its adequate response variability. One point should be made clear; services that treat patients with respiratory disorders, mainly associated with pulmonary hypertension, should have inhaled NO as a therapeutic resource. In the absence of trials involving a larger number of patients, and despite its toxic potential, inhaled NO should be used with extreme technical rigor, as a therapeutic test that can save lives.

Possible Use of Nitric Oxide as a Complimentary Therapeutic Measure in Distributive Circulatory Shock

As it is gas, NO enters the lungs and is deactivated by binding to hemoglobin in the pulmonary circulation, and its vasodilatory action does not reach peripheral regions outside the lungs. The selective NO vasodilation on pulmonary vessels is what currently makes its inhalation one of the primary therapeutic resources for pulmonary hypertension control. However, it has become a collective experience to discover that NO inhalation is not as effective when associated with sepsis. One reason for this is probably the systemic arterial hypotension produced by sepsis when no therapy is effective, and there is no response to vasopressors, a situation in which the prognosis is poor. The use of nitric oxide synthase (NOS) inhibitors against low blood pressure, resulting from excessive NO production, would be a logical idea. Initially, good results were reported in animal experiments with NOS inhibitors only. However, it was observed that the administration of NOS inhibitors carries a considerable risk of decreasing cardiac output and tissue blood flow or myocardial ischemia. Thus, this has recently been considered an inappropriate treatment [1].

On the other hand, it has been shown in animal experiments that pulmonary hypertension is a complication with endotoxemia. Therefore, it makes it possible to adopt a treatment strategy that targets pulmonary hypertension, in addition to systemic arterial hypotension. Relatively positive results have been reported in studies of combination therapy with synthetic NOS inhibitors to treat systemic arterial hypotension and inhalation NO to treat pulmonary hypertension [1].

The cause of pulmonary hypertension in a state of septicemic shock is probably multifactorial. These factors possibly include thromboxane, perivascular edema, intravascular obstruction, and hypoxic vasoconstriction. Currently, the NO role in septic pulmonary hypertension is not clearly understood. However, as only pulmonary arteries are constricted, the release of some type of vasoconstrictor is not likely, and there appears to be some side effect of hypoxia because of the degrading condition. Therefore, the endotoxin shock is expressed as an increase in pulmonary vascular resistance (PVR) and a decrease in systemic vascular resistance (SVR). As in the treatment of endotoxic shock, NO inhalation and NOS inhibition are related to the risk of complications. NO reacts readily with oxygen, leading to NO formation, which is an irritant of the airways, and in higher concentrations, it can produce severe lung damage. Also, NO in the reaction with hemoglobin leads to the formation of methemoglobin, which, if accumulated, can lead to anemic hypoxia. It has been shown that NO inhalation can prolong bleeding time in healthy individuals, an effect that should be considered in the treatment of septic patients, whose coagulation system is frequently affected. NO inhalation alone has proven to be beneficial in the treatment of pulmonary hypertension of different genesis but needs further investigation on toxicology and outcome [8–12].

Concluding Remarks

- The treatment effectiveness in isolated cases.
- The therapeutic response variability regardless of age, heart, or respiratory disease.
- Better therapeutic intervention, albeit transitory, in cases of more severe and chronic pulmonary hypertension.
- The belief that inhaled NO would be a potential therapeutic weapon in transient hypertension; thus, neonatology and cardiopulmonary transplants could be benefited.
- Everyone was apprehensive about the potential NO toxicity, not only for patients but also for professionals who used it.
- It seems that, in more than a decade, these observations are still current and pertinent. Only a consensus appears to be established, namely, the use of smaller doses (10–20 ppm) than those initially used.

References

1. Tavares AP, Pimenta Junior AG, Evora PR. [Basis for the therapeutic use of inhaled nitric oxide]. Arq Bras Cardiol. 1995;64(1):45–52.
2. Morris K, Beghetti M, Petros A, Adatia I, Bohn D. Comparison of hyperventilation and inhaled nitric oxide for pulmonary hypertension after repair of congenital heart disease. Crit Care Med. 2000;28(8):2974–8.
3. Allman KG, Young JD, Carapiet D, Stevens JE, Ostman-Smith I, Archer LN. Effects of oxygen and nitric oxide in oxygen on pulmonary arterial pressures of children with congenital cardiac defects. Pediatr Cardiol. 1996;17(4):246–50.
4. Sharma R, Raizada N, Choudhary SK, Bhan A, Kumar P, Juneja R, et al. Does inhaled nitric oxide improve survival in operated congenital disease with severe pulmonary hypertension? Indian Heart J. 2001;53(1):48–55.
5. Curran RD, Mavroudis C, Backer CL, Sautel M, Zales VR, Wessel DL. Inhaled nitric oxide for children with congenital heart disease and pulmonary hypertension. Ann Thorac Surg. 1995;60(6):1765–71.
6. Laitinen PO, Rasanen J, Sairanen H. Postoperative nitric oxide therapy in children with congenital heart disease. Can the need be predicted? Scand Cardiovasc J. 2000;34(2):149–53.
7. Ichida F, Uese K, Hashimoto I, Hamamichi Y, Tsubata S, Fukahara K, et al. Acute effect of oral prostacyclin and inhaled nitric oxide on pulmonary hypertension in children. J Cardiol. 1997;29(4):217–24.
8. Rimensberger PC, Spahr-Schopfer I, Berner M, Jaeggi E, Kalangos A, Friedli B, et al. Inhaled nitric oxide versus aerosolized iloprost in secondary pulmonary hypertension in children with congenital heart disease: vasodilator capacity and cellular mechanisms. Circulation. 2001;103(4):544–8.

9. Ivy DD, Kinsella JP, Ziegler JW, Abman SH. Dipyridamole attenuates rebound pulmonary hypertension after inhaled nitric oxide withdrawal in postoperative congenital heart disease. J Thorac Cardiovasc Surg. 1998;115(4):875–82.

10. Yahagi N, Kumon K, Tanigami H, Watanabe Y, Haruna M, Hayashi H, et al. Cardiac surgery and inhaled nitric oxide: indication and follow-up (2-4 years). Artif Organs. 1998;22(10):886–91.

11. Atz AM, Wessel DL. Nitric oxide inhalation. In: Rubanyi GM, editor. Pathophysiology and clinical applications of nitric oxide. Netherlands: Harwood Academic Publishers; 1999. p. 471–503.

12. Omar HA, Gong F, Sun MY, Einzig S. Nebulized nitroglycerin in children with pulmonary hypertension secondary to congenital heart disease. W V Med J. 1999;95(2):74–5.

Index

Printed in the United States
by Baker & Taylor Publisher Services